Topics in Trauma Surgery

Edited by Selim Sözen

Published in London, United Kingdom

Topics in Trauma Surgery
http://dx.doi.org/10.5772/intechopen.105335
Edited by Selim Sözen

Contributors
Leighton J. Reynolds, Ashok Kumar Puranik, Althea Vency Cardoz, Andrey Semenov, Dmitriy Vybornov, Nikolaj Tarasov, Vladimir Krestyashin, Vladimir Koroteev, Ivan Isaev, Alberto Jorge-Mora, Jesús Pino-Mínguez, Alberto De Castro, Samer Amhaz-Escanlar, Renzo Reyes, Mohammad Meshkini, José Miguel Aceves-Ayala, David Jacob Álvarez-Chávez, Clara Elizabeth Valdez-Cruz, Cristhian Felipe Montoya-Salazar, Carlos Alfredo Bautista-López, Cesar Alberto Ortiz-Orozco, Wence Francisco Villalvazo-Zuñiga, Pablo Francisco Rojas-Solís, Selim Sözen, Emrah Şahin, İlhan Bali, Muhammed Said Dalkılıç, Mehmet Gençtürk, Merih Yilmaz, Burhan Hakan Kanat

First published in London, United Kingdom, 2023 by IntechOpen
IntechOpen is the global imprint of INTECHOPEN LIMITED, registered in England and Wales, registration number: 11086078, 5 Princes Gate Court, London, SW7 2QJ, United Kingdom

British Library Cataloguing-in-Publication Data
A catalogue record for this book is available from the British Library

Additional hard and PDF copies can be obtained from orders@intechopen.com

Topics in Trauma Surgery
Edited by Selim Sözen
p. cm.
Print ISBN 978-1-83768-438-0
Online ISBN 978-1-83768-439-7
eBook (PDF) ISBN 978-1-83768-440-3

Meet the editor

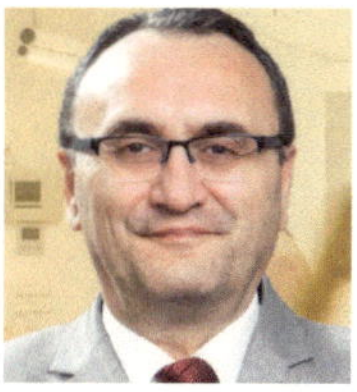

Dr. Selim Sözen is an expert in general surgery who received his medical degree from Ondokuz Mayıs University, Turkey, in 1998. From 1999 to 2004, he was an assistant doctor at Ankara Atatürk Education and Research Hospital, Turkey. From 2004 to 2013, he worked as a specialist at different government hospitals in Turkey. He joined the Department of General Surgery, Medicine Faculty, Namık Kemal University, Turkey, as an associate professor in 2013. He completed liver transplantation surgery at İnönü University, Turkey, in 2014–2015. Since 2016, Dr. Sözen has run his own surgery clinic in İstanbul, Turkey. He is a member of the Turkish Surgical Association and a review board member for several journals. He has published 105 articles in scientific journals and presented 64 poster papers at scientific congresses. His research interests include general, gastrointestinal, emergency, and trauma surgery, bacterial translocation, liver disease, and hernia surgery.

Contents

Preface IX

Section 1
Clinical Cases 1

Chapter 1 3
Abdominal Trauma
by Emrah Şahin, İlhan Bali, Muhammed Said Dalkiliç, Mehmet Gençtürk, Merih Yilmaz, Burhan Hakan Kanat and Selim Sözen

Chapter 2 19
Appropriate Protective Measures for the Prevention of Animal-related Goring Injuries
by Ashok Kumar Puranik and Althea Vency Cardoz

Chapter 3 31
Management of Duodenal Injuries
by José Miguel Aceves-Ayala, David Jacob Álvarez-Chávez, Clara Elizabeth Valdez-Cruz, Cristhian Felipe Montoya-Salazar, Carlos Alfredo Bautista-López, Cesar Alberto Ortiz-Orozco, Wence Francisco Villalvazo-Zuñiga and Pablo Francisco Rojas-Solís

Chapter 4 41
Ultrasound Empowered Trauma Management
by Mohammad Meshkini

Chapter 5 61
OCD of the Knee in Adolescents
by Andrey Semenov, Dmitriy Vybornov, Nikolaj Tarasov, Vladimir Krestyashin, Ivan Isaev and Vladimir Koroteev

Chapter 6 89
Distal Femoral Fractures
by Renzo Reyes, María González-Alonso, Samer Amhaz-Escanlar, Alberto De Castro, Jesús Pino-Mínguez and Alberto Jorge-Mora

Section 2
New Perspectives **105**

Chapter 7 **107**
Perspective Chapter: "The Complex Architecture of a Traumatic Brain Injury"
by Leighton J. Reynolds

Preface

This book is a collection of chapters on trauma surgery. It is divided into two sections with chapters focusing on different clinical specialties.

In Section 1, Chapter 1, "Abdominal Trauma," Sözen et al. discuss abdominal trauma.

Chapter 2, "Appropriate Protective Measures for the Prevention of Animal-related Goring Injuries" by Ashok Kumar Puranik and Althea Vency Cardoz discusses the types and treatment of animal attack injuries. Animal attack injuries are seen all over the world. Other than a few case reports and case series, this mode of injury is highly underreported. Hence, the global burden of animal attack injuries is unknown.

Chapter 3, "Management of Duodenal Injuries" by José Miguel Aceves-Ayala et al., examines duodenal injuries and their importance.

Chapter 4, "Ultrasound-Empowered Trauma Management" by Mohammad Meshkini, emphasizes the importance of using ultrasonography in trauma patients.

Chapter 5, "OCD of the Knee in Adolescents" by Andrey Semenov et al., focuses on osteochondritis dissecans (OCD) of the knee. The last stage of OCD is the separation of the osteochondral fragment, leaving a full-thickness osteochondral defect that is usually filled with low-quality fibrocartilaginous tissue. This tissue provides weak resistance to peak loading forces, which puts the patient at risk of further destruction of the subchondral bone and the development of early osteoarthritis.

Chapter 6, "Distal Femoral Fractures" by Alberto Jorge-Mora et al., discusses new techniques for treating femoral fractures in elderly and younger patients.

In Section 2, Chapter 7, "Perspective Chapter: The Complex Architecture of a Traumatic Brain Injury", Leighton J. Reynolds draws attention to traumatic brain injuries from different points of view.

I thank the authors for their professional dedication and outstanding work in summarizing their clinical and research practices.

Selim Sözen
Associate Professor of General Surgery,
Sözen Surgery Clinic,
Tekirdağ, Turkey

Section 1

Clinical Cases

Chapter 1

Abdominal Trauma

Emrah Şahin, İlhan Bali, Muhammed Said Dalkiliç, Mehmet Gençtürk, Merih Yilmaz, Burhan Hakan Kanat and Selim Sözen

Abstract

Abdominal trauma accounts for 7–10% of hospital admissions due to trauma. Depending on the mechanism of occurrence, abdominal traumas are classified as either blunt or penetrating. The most important risk after trauma is hypovolemic shock. Deaths caused by blunt trauma are frequently the result of diagnostic difficulties and treatment delays. Abdominal surgery after traumatic injury is performed for two reasons; bleeding due to injury to vascular structures or a solid organ (e.g., spleen, liver, kidney) or injury due to perforation of a hollow organ (stomach, small intestine, colon, gallbladder). Patients may remain asymptomatic until they have lost 50–60% of their blood volume. Through inspection, auscultation, and palpation, the damaged organs and the presence of hemorrhage should be examined during the physical examination. The findings of peritoneal irritation are incredibly critical. Even though some studies indicate a mortality rate as high as 25.8% for abdominal injuries, the overall mortality rate is 10%. Other studies reveal mortality rates ranging from 15% to 17.1%. It should not be forgotten that the patient with abdominal trauma may have multi-trauma. The patient's vital signs, abdominal examination, and hematocrit should be checked at frequent intervals. Early surgical evaluation is important. It is important to remember that the main source of bleeding and shock may be the abdomen.

Keywords: abdominal trauma, hemorrhage, hypovolemic shock, blunt trauma, diagnostic laparoscopy

1. Introduction

Abdominal trauma accounts for 7–10% of hospital admissions due to trauma. In people under the age of 45, 10% of trauma-related deaths are caused by abdominal trauma [1].

Motor vehicle accidents, abdominal blows, and falls account for the majority of abdominal injuries. Less common causes of abdominal trauma include penetrating injuries, home accidents, and iatrogenic conditions [2].

Depending on the mechanism of occurrence, abdominal traumas are classified as either blunt or penetrating. Blunt abdominal injuries are seen in approximately three quarters of the patients [3]. In some studies, it has been reported that the most common abdominal injury is penetrating injury [4]. Most blunt abdominal traumas occur after motor vehicle accidents. It is usually accompanied by multitrauma. The most important risk after trauma is hypovolemic shock. Deaths caused by blunt trauma are frequently the result of diagnostic difficulties and treatment delays.

Typically, a penetrating injury is caused by violence, such as a stab wound or gunshot wound. Gunshot wounds result from the explosion effect (a combination of blunt and penetrating trauma associated with blasts). The causes of penetrating abdominal injuries include accidental, homicidal, iatrogenic, and gunshot wounds [2].

Abdominal surgery after traumatic injury is performed for two reasons; bleeding due to injury to vascular structures or a solid organ (e.g., spleen, liver, kidney) or injury due to perforation of a hollow organ (stomach, small intestine, colon, gallbladder).

The first intervention of trauma patients prior to arrival at the hospital is crucial for clinical outcomes [5]. It has been demonstrated that a delay in trauma patients' arrival at the hospital significantly increases their risk of morbidity and mortality [6].

Almost all deaths are mostly caused by bleeding that occurs immediately after injury. In the late stage, it is related to septic complications [7].

Although many trauma patients do not require immediate laparotomy, emergency surgery should be considered in patients with suspected intra-abdominal injury and who are hemodynamically unstable.

Patients who are hemodynamically stable should usually undergo further diagnostic investigations such as abdominal computed tomography (CT) scanning. Sometimes, these patients are treated in interventional radiology units with diagnostic angiography followed by therapeutic embolization when CT shows the possibility of arterial extravasation.

Nonsurgical Conservative treatment experience is mostly based on blunt abdominal trauma experience. Some publications also state that nonoperative treatment of gunshot and stab wounds can be performed in selected patients [8, 9].

In the past decade, the concept of "damage control" has revolutionized surgical practice by restricting early therapeutic procedures to those required to achieve hemostasis and deferring reconstructive surgeries such as intestinal anastomoses until enough resuscitation is achieved [10].

Surgery can be delayed if the patient is hemodynamically stable and requires an examination to identify other system injuries (nervous system, bone, thoracic, and vascular) [10].

2. Classification: types of trauma

Traumas can be blunt, penetrating, or blunt-penetrating (mixed) based on their mechanism; thus, the affected organs can vary. Depending on the location of the trauma, one or more internal organs may be damaged.

1. *Blunt traumas*: It is mostly caused by motor vehicle accidents, beating, or falling from a height. In this type of trauma, the mechanisms of injury are direct blow (pressure), crushing (compression), or deceleration (rupture). The organs most commonly affected are the spleen, small intestine, and liver [11].

2. *Penetrating traumas*: Penetrating traumas consist of stab wounds and gunshot wounds.

Stab wounds: Penetrating tools cause low-energy penetrating injuries. The mechanism of injury is tear-cut, and the liver, small intestine, diaphragm, and colon are most commonly affected. In peritoneal penetration, a physical examination, diagnostic peritoneal lavage (DPL), and local exploration are required. A laparotomy may be needed if the diagnosis cannot be confirmed.

Gunshot wounds: High-energy injuries occur in penetrating traumas due to gunshot wounds (GSW). The mechanism of injury can be cavitation, disruption, and fragmentation. Small intestine, colon, liver, and vascular structures are most commonly affected in GSW-related injuries. Peritoneal penetration is important and requires laparotomy. CT with contrast is recommended for back and flank injuries. In cases with single entry, abdominal X-ray graphics can be helpful in identifying traces. It is difficult to determine the trace in multiple entries [12, 13].

3. *Mixed traumas*: There are both penetrating and blunt traumas(**Figures 1** and **2**).

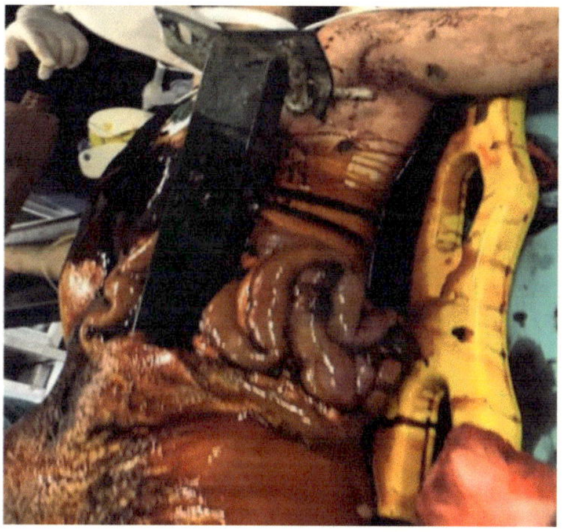

Figure 1.
Falling from height, multiple small and large intestine, rectum, anal sphincter, bladder, prostate injury. Trauma-related bladder and prostate were completely absent. There were hematomas and perforation in the small intestine and large bowel. Small bowel resection and anastomosis were performed. Performed left-end colostomy for anal region and rectum injury. Permanent urostomy performed for bladder injury (absence).

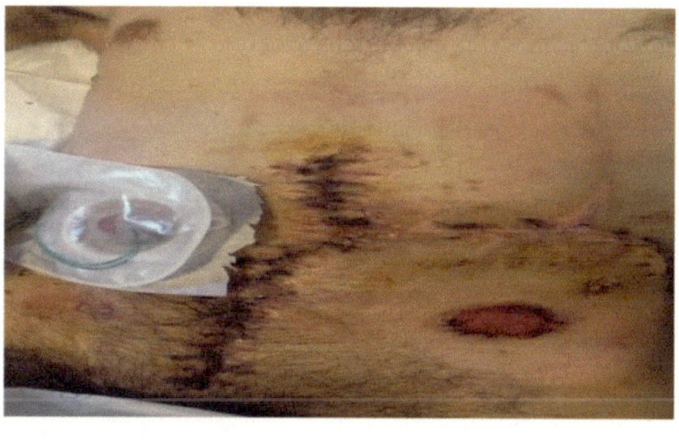

Figure 2.
Right permanent urostomy, left colostomy.

3. Clinical presentation

There is an insidious clinical picture. Patients may remain asymptomatic until they have lost 50–60% of their blood volume. It is frequently overlooked under conditions that alter the neurologic picture, such as head trauma and alcohol consumption.

Until there is significant intra-abdominal blood loss, abdominal pain and distension may not occur. More than 35% of patients initially exhibit normal vital signs and examinations despite the presence of severe intra-abdominal hemorrhage.

4. Priorities

Initial evaluation should focus on intra-abdominal hemorrhage and shock. When abnormal vital signs are seen, shock and hemorrhage should be investigated. The possibility of occult intra-abdominal injury is an indication of laparotomy.

5. Physical examination

The abdomen should be checked comprehensively for any signs of injury. Head trauma, spinal cord injury, multi-trauma, altered consciousness, mental retardation, pregnancy, and old age all contribute to an unreliable physical examination. Especially in such conflicting conditions, repeated and thorough examinations are essential. It must be performed every 30 minutes for the first four hours, then every two to four hours thereafter.

Through inspection, auscultation, and palpation, the damaged organs and the presence of hemorrhage should be examined during the physical examination. The findings of peritoneal irritation are incredibly critical.

In the inspection process, finds are explored for using the *CLAP* algorithm: contusion, laseration, abrasion, and penetration.

Intestinal sounds should be listened to for a least one minute during auscultation. If rigidity and perioneal irritation are present, bowel sounds are either absent or weak.

On palpation, the presence of distension is first evaluated. It is assessed based on defense, rebound, and rigidity. The most painful portion is left for last, and the abdomen is palpated. On palpation, the legs must be drawn toward the abdomen.

The examination of pelvic instability, genital examination, rectal examination, and back and vertebral examination should be done.

The fundamental principle in abdominal trauma is to stabilize the patient and prioritize interventions to accomplish this.

Findings leading to the diagnosis should be carefully examined. The presence of gross hematuria, hypotension, lower rib fractures, hemothorax or pneumothorax, abdominal abrasions, or hematomas gives an idea about the organs likely to be injured [14].

Despite physical examination and imaging, retroperitoneal injuries, pancreatic injuries, mesenteric injuries, hollow organ injuries, and urinary injuries can be overlooked.

5.1 Laboratory tests

The patient's blood group and cross-match, hemoglobin and hematocrit, PT, aPTT, and INR levels should be measured to reduce the risk of hemorrhage.

6. Diagnostic techniques

Direct radiography, ultrasonography (USG), computed Tomography (CT), diagnostic peritoneal lavage (DPL), diagnostic laparoscopy, angiography, and diagnostic peritoneal lavage.

6.1 Direct graphy

Standing direct abdominal and PA chest radiographs have limited utility in cases of abdominal trauma. They may be useful in the presence of concomitant thoracic trauma. They can be particularly useful in locating foreign names or lead fragments. Pelvic X-ray can be seen in a suspected pelvic fracture.

6.2 Ultrasonography (USG): Focused assessment with sonography for trauma (FAST)

It is non-invasive, highly sensitive, inexpensive, and mobile. The fact that it can be applied even in unstable patients and can diagnose at the bedside makes it an advantageous method. It is the best technique for the diagnosis of intra-abdominal bleeding in trauma patients. Identify solid organ injuries. It should be done twice with an interval of at least 6 hours. Repeated FAST increases sensitivity in diagnosis.

In the initial evaluation of trauma patients, FAST should be performed on all patients, if possible. In the FAST technique, free fluid in the abdomen is investigated in the areas listed below.

- Subxiphoid view (Pericardial fluid)
- Right upper quadrant (Morisson pouch)
- Left upper quadrant (Splenorenal space)
- Pelvic view (Douglas/Rectovesical pouch)

However, USG is not an appropriate method in the evaluation of bowel perforation. It is also insufficient in terms of evaluating the retroperitoneal area.

6.3 Computed tomography (CT)

It is a suitable imaging method for stable trauma patients. Today, CT has become the gold standard in the evaluation of abdominal trauma. Intravenous contrast-enhanced imaging allows evaluation of both the peritoneal cavity and the retroperitoneum. It also allows the assessment of the duodenum and pancreas, extravasation from the ureter, and the amount of blood in the abdomen. It may also show additional injuries, but it is insufficient to detect hollow organ injuries [15].

The sensitivity for intra-abdominal injury was 95%, and the specificity was 97%. It is very useful and successful in retroperitoneal organ injuries. The sensitivity and specificity in cases of bowel and mesenteric trauma were, respectively, 94% and 96% [16].

It is not successful in the initial stage of pancreatic injuries. It can identify the patients who will result an operational decision in liver and spleen injuries. Intestinal, diaphragm, and pancreatic injuries may not be recognized. In addition, it is useful for detecting retroperitoneal hemorrhage.

6.4 Diagnostic peritoneal lavage (DPL)

Because of CT and USG, it is no longer the first choice method in the evaluation of hemoperitoneum. It is 100% sensitive and 83% specific for hemoperitoneum. The major complication rate is 1% [17, 18]. If the clinical condition of the patient does not allow for examinations such as CT or USG, DPL may be preferred.

6.5 Angiography

It is not a routinely used option. Angiography can show intraparenchymal vascular injuries and active bleeding in the abdominal organs. It can be useful in pelvic traumas. Bleeding in the spleen, liver, and retroperitoneum can be treated with embolization and angiography without the need for surgery.

6.6 Emergency laparotomy

Emergency laparotomy should be performed when the patient's hemodynamic status does not improve with initial resuscitation, peritoneal irritation findings are present, peritoneal penetration of abdominal injury with gunshot, bile and intestinal contents are present in the DPL, and the patient has evisceration.

Laparotomy is indicated in the presence of abnormal vital signs such as tachycardia and hypotension after blunt abdominal trauma, signs of shock without blood loss, signs of peritonitis, and the presence of additional injuries (such as lower rib fracture).

Emergency surgery should be performed in cases of external bleeding accompanied by hypotension and shock after penetrating injuries, positive peritoneal lavage, subsequent deterioration of consciousness, and sudden abdominal distension.

Emergency laparotomy should be performed if extraluminal air is detected on direct X-ray, diaphragmatic rupture is detected, amylase elevation accompanying positive physical examination findings in the abdomen, intraperitoneal bladder rupture, blood in the nasogastric drainage or rectal examination is detected.

Emergency laparotomy should be performed in the presence of fluid during FAST, positive DPL, contrast extravasation or extraluminal air on gastrointestinal radiological images, severe pelvis fracture, bladder rupture on a contrast cystogram, or gross hematuria.

Laparoscopy can be used for the diagnosis and treatment of blunt and penetrating traumas [19]. Diagnostic and therapeutic laparoscopy is recommended in blunt abdominal trauma for diaphragmatic injury, mesenteric injury, hollow organ injury, and in cases where the patient's clinical condition is unstable [20].

7. Trauma-related organ injuries

The abdomen is divided into three regions: the peritoneal cavity, the pelvis, and the retroperitoneal space. The upper peritoneal cavity contains the diaphragm, liver, spleen, stomach, and colon, whereas the lower peritoneal cavity contains the small intestine and colon.

The retroperitoneal space contains the aorta, vena cava, pancreas, duodenum, and ureters. There are structures such as the rectum, bladder, uterus, and iliac vessels in the pelvis.

7.1 Solid organ injuries

Liver, spleen, pancreas, kidney, diaphragm, and abdominal wall injuries.

Trauma to solid organs causes symptoms related to bleeding. Vital signs and hypotension may develop rapidly. As a result of progressive blood loss, tachycardia, skin changes, and changes in consciousness can be seen. With severe intra-abdominal damage, abdominal tenderness, distention, and tympanism may occur later. The risk of mortality and morbidity due to blood loss is high.

7.2 Hollow organ injuries

Stomach, duodenum, small intestine, colon, rectum, gallbladder, bile ducts, and genitourinary system injuries.

Due to the bacterial content in the small intestine and colon, inflammation develops within hours. This can cause septic conditions due to bleeding and peritoneal contamination (**Figure 3**).

7.3 Retroperitoneal injuries

Retroperitoneal injuries are often initially asymptomatic. Diagnosis can be difficult due to their location and limitation of symptoms. Nausea, vomiting, abdominal

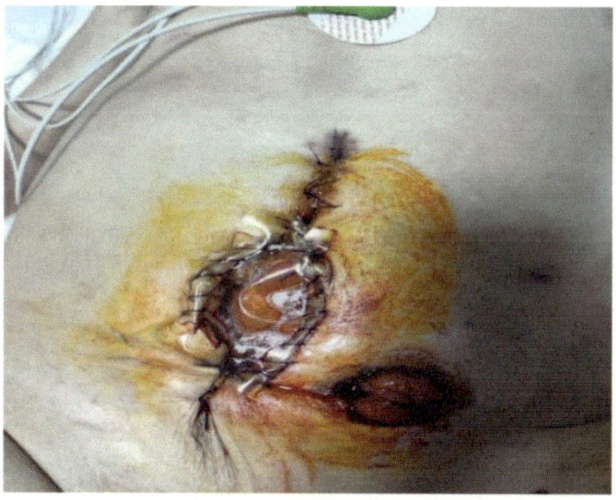

Figure 3.
Small bowel and colon perforation due to blunt abdominal trauma in an elderly patient. Small bowel resection, double barrel ostomy (colostomy), and Bogota bag technique. Since the intra-abdominal pressure will increase when the abdomen is closed, the Bogota bag technique, which is a temporary closure method, maybe a good alternative [21].

pain, and fever may develop in duodenal injuries. Diagnosis is difficult in pancreatic injury, increased amylase supports the diagnosis. It may initially appear normal on CT imaging. Retroperitoneal injuries occur more frequently after being hit by high-speed vehicles or falling from a height.

7.4 Esophageal injury

Blunt or penetrating trauma of the esophagus is rare. There are symptoms such as severe chest pain and fever, bloody vomiting, dysphagia, and respiratory distress after hours.

Diagnosis is made by finding air in the mediastinum, pleural effusion or hydropneumothorax on endoscopy or radiological imaging.

Treatment options include wound debridement, suture repair, drainage, and esophageal diversion in delayed cases.

7.5 Stomach injury

The stomach is resistant to blunt injuries. Most are due to penetrating trauma to the epigastric region. Vascular support is quite high. Bleeding from the nasogastric tube suggests a gastric injury.

The gastrocolic omentum should be opened widely. Debridement is done as needed. The outcomes of primary repair are excellent.

7.6 Duodenum injury

Since it is located retroperitoneally, it is usually diagnosed after laparotomy. Signs and symptoms may develop late. Duodenum injury indicates severe trauma. Mortality increases up to 4 times in delayed cases.

Serum amylase may be elevated. Radiograph shows retroperitoneal air. Diagnosis is made with oral and intravenous contrast-enhanced CT. Laparotomy is mandatory.

7.7 Small intestine injury

The incidence of small bowel injury in penetrating abdominal trauma reaches up to 50%. This rate is 5–15% in blunt traumas. In most cases, signs of peritoneal irritation due to injury are seen. Relatively less mobile segments, such as the jejunum near the ligament of Treitz and the distal ileum near the ileocecal valve, are more susceptible to injury. Mesenteric injuries range from simple contusions to mesenteric avulsions. In cases where only vascular structures are injured, symptoms may be delayed until bowel ischemia develops.

Free air can be visualized by direct graphy. USG can show even a very small amount of free fluid.

In most cases, debridement and primary repair are sufficient. Simple incisions are repaired with "Lembert" sutures. Resection and anastomosis should be preferred if the damage to the intestinal wall is extensive or if there are multiple perforation foci that are close to each other. Due to the adequate vascular supply, the surgical outcomes are satisfactory.

7.8 Colon injury

Delaying surgery increases the risk of increased contamination. Classical treatment involved the creation of a proximal diverting colostomy with bowel repair or conversion of the injured area to a colostomy. Today, the routine creation of a colostomy is contradictory. Primary repair can be performed in right colon injuries with minimal contamination. Colostomies can be created in right colon injuries with severe contamination or in severe left colon injuries. Surgical site infection due to bowel injury is the most common postoperative complication. IntestinalDue to the bacterial content, suppurative peritonitis symptoms may occur from 6 to 8 hours after injury. Contents leak into the peritoneal cavity, contaminating the peritoneal cavity (and thus the surgical wound) with intestinal bacteria [22]. Due to the bacterial content, symptoms indicating suppurative peritonitis may appear 6–8 hours after injury.

7.9 Rectum injury

Since it is a retroperitoneal organ, the diagnosis may be difficult, but the symptoms are indistinct. Rectal injury should be suspected in pelvic fractures. Early diagnosis and treatment provide reduced mortality and morbidity. If the injury is full thickness and above the dentate line, primary repair is not performed without a colostomy. In most cases, an end sigmoid colostomy is created proximal to the injury, the distal rectum is irrigated with saline solution, and drains are implanted. For injuries below the dentate line, debridement and primary repair and drainage are sufficient without colonic diversion.

8. Injury of the gallbladder and biliary tracts

Among abdominal traumas, gallbladder injuries are relatively rare. It is usually associated with penetrating trauma and liver injuries [23].

USG is the first examination in the imaging of the biliary tract. Intra-abdominal collection can be detected. Bile leakage and fistulas can be detected by MRCP examination using liver-specific contrast material. Leakage and fistula can be easily demonstrated on images taken in the biliary phase [2]. The treatment is cholecystectomy. In blunt trauma, common bile duct injury may also occur with papilla rupture. These types of injuries are difficult to diagnose before surgery. If necessary, an intraoperative cholangiogram should be taken, and careful exploration should be performed.

8.1 Liver injury

Isolated injuries are rare and are associated with other organ injuries in 70–90% of cases [2]. The liver is the most frequently injured organ in blunt and penetrating abdominal trauma [24].

Ultrasonography (USG) is the first imaging method in cases with stable general conditions. USG shows intra-abdominal fluid collections and parenchymal lesions. A positive USG finding is an indication of CT. Bleeding cannot be detected when more than 50% of liver injuries are explored. Bleeding can be stopped with primary sutures, cautery, or hemostatic agents. Mortality is over 50% in massive traumas associated with vena cava or hepatic vein injury. Thanks to CT examination, lesions that can be treated without surgery can be recognized. In many studies, the failure rate in non-surgical follow-up is less than 10% (**Figure 4**) [24].

8.2 Spleen injury

The spleen is the most frequently injured intra-abdominal organ in blunt trauma. Due to its cancellous structure, it is sensitive to trauma and is responsible for significant bleeding. It is often associated with other organ injuries. The main symptoms are tachycardia, hypotension, and syncope due to blood loss. Left shoulder pain (Kehr's sign) is the classic finding of spleen injuries. There is tenderness and pain in the left upper quadrant. Fractures in the lower ribs should suggest injury to the spleen. After clamping the splenic artery, blood pressure usually stabilizes. CT has a sensitivity and specificity of up to 95% for spleen injuries [2].

The classical treatment method is splenectomy. With the high incidence of sepsis after splenectomy, more selective approaches are now preferred, and splenic repair and nonoperative follow-up are among the treatment options [26]. From 60% to 90% of patients with spleen injuries are conservatively treated [27]. Polyvalent pneumococcal vaccine is administered after splenectomy.

8.3 Pancreatic injury

Although pancreatic injuries are rare, mortality and morbidity rates are high. Isolated pancreatic injury is rare and does not usually lead to massive bleeding. It is most commonly seen with duodenal injuries in penetrating traumas. Imaging findings may be negative in the first 12 hours after trauma. Mortality and morbidity are very high due to autodigestion caused by exocrine secretions in delayed diagnosis and treatment [2, 23]. Damage to the pancreatic duct is crucial and requires operative treatment, including control of bleeding, resection, and drainage of necrotic or damaged pancreatic tissue. CT is very useful in diagnosis. Endoscopic retrograde

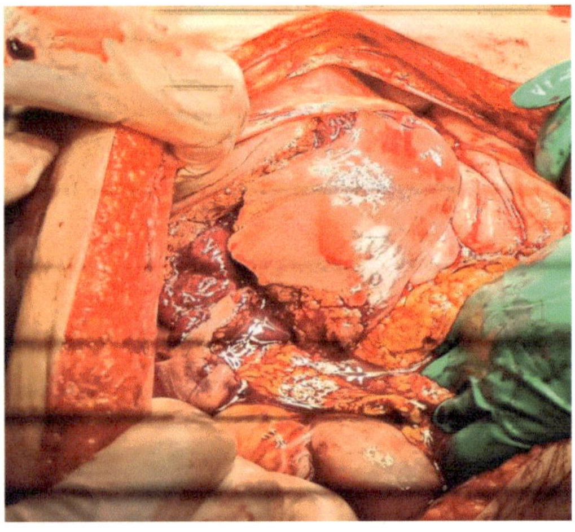

Figure 4.
Blunt abdominal trauma involving segment 5,6,7,8 and large branches of the middle hepatic vein injuries. Large branches of the middle hepatic vein suturing and perihepatic packing. Removing of liver packs 36 hours after insertion reduced the risk of rebleeding [25].

cholangiopancreatography (ERCP) is the gold standard for both diagnosis and treatment. Pseudocyst can be seen as a late complication.

8.4 Kidney injury

Approximately 10% of blunt abdominal traumas result in kidney injury. Lower rib fractures, thoracolumbar injury, macroscopic hematuria, and hypotension with microscopic hematuria should be evaluated for renal trauma in blunt trauma. The kidney is the most frequently injured part of the urinary tract [2].

Hematuria is present in 90–95% of cases. Macroscopic hematuria often accompanies severe trauma. If there is a ureteral tear, vascular pedicle injury, or ureteropelvic junction avulsion, hematuria may not be present. Complications such as urinary extravasation, urinoma, hemorrhage, perirenal abscess, pseudoaneurysm, hypertension, and arteriovenous fistula can be seen. Renovascular hypertension may develop as a result of prolonged compression of the renal parenchyma by subcapsular hematoma or urinoma [2].

Renal bleeding itself is rarely the cause of hemodynamic instability. It is usually followed up with non-surgical treatment. Continued bleeding, Gerota's fascia injury, or renal function loss require surgery. Diagnosis can be made with contrast-enhanced CT, and cystography.

9. Genitourinary system injury

The ureter is the least injured part of the urinary tract and is usually penetrating injuries of iatrogenic origin. There is no hematuria in 1/3 of the cases. Ureteral injuries can easily be overlooked and cases may present with late complications such as urinoma, periureteral abscess, fistula, and stenosis [2].

Blunt, penetrating, or iatrogenic injuries of the bladder may occur. Bladder rupture is a common form of injury. Hematuria is observed in bladder injury. Pelvic fracture is present in almost all cases of bladder injury [2, 23]. Because the urine is sterile, peritoneal symptoms may only be observed in bladder perforation cases. Minor injuries may spontaneously heal within one to two weeks. Major injuries require surgical intervention. Urine output is reduced or absent in perforations. As a result of the resorption of urine from the peritoneum, urea increases in the blood [2].

10. Diaphragmatic injuries

Diaphragmatic injuries are usually diagnosed late as they do not cause obvious symptoms. Abdominal organs seen in the thorax on direct thorax should be suspected in case of pleural effusion. Diagnosis can be made with CT, MRI, thoracoscopy, and laparoscopy. Herniation can occur months or years after injury. Treatment is surgery.

11. Abdominal wall injuries

There is a risk of evisceration in penetrating injuries of the abdominal wall. Rectus hematoma is the most common form of injury. Since there is a possibility of multiple injuries in many abdominal organs in these patients, surgery is performed without the need for DPL. First, the comorbid injuries and then the abdominal wall injury is addressed.

12. Injury to vascular structures

Both artery and vein injuries in the abdomen are life-threatening. Controlling both proximal and distal parts should be the main principle.

Solid organ damage can result in massive bleeding and hypovolemia. The primary complication of injury to hollow organs is abdominal or systemic sepsis. Failure to find anything in the laparotomy does not mean that the laparotomy was performed incorrectly.

13. General approach to abdominal trauma

1. Investigate any intra-abdominal bleeding.

2. Fix unstable vital signs due to shock and bleeding.

3. Determine if the source of bleeding is in the abdomen.

4. Decide if an urgent laparotomy is needed.

5. Thorough examination, laboratory, and radiological tests to determine if there is an occult intra-abdominal injury.

6. Monitor the patient with frequent physical examinations.

The causes of abdominal injuries vary by country. Most abdominal injuries in Europe are blunt trauma from traffic accidents. Gunshot wounds to the abdomen are the most common cause in Africa [28]. Although motor vehicle accidents are an important social problem in our country, stab injuries constitute the majority of abdominal injuries in our clinics. Most thoracic abdominal injuries are associated with other parts of the body such as the chest and limbs. Hemodynamic instability, chest and extremity injuries, and abdominal trauma should be questioned in patients with low Glasgow scores.

14. Conclusion

Although some studies put the mortality rate of abdominal injuries as high as 25.8%, the overall mortality rate is 10% [29]. However, some other studies reveal that mortality rates vary between 15% and 17.1% [3, 22].

It should not be forgotten that the patient with abdominal trauma may have multi-trauma. The patient's vital signs, abdominal examination, and hematocrit should be checked at frequent intervals. Early surgical evaluation is important. It is important to remember that the main source of bleeding and shock may be the abdomen.

Nonoperative treatment can be applied in hemodynamically stable blunt abdominal trauma patients with normal physical examination findings [29]. Similarly, hemodynamically stable patients with penetrating injuries can be treated non-operatively in the absence of symptoms of peritonitis. These patients should be followed up with close clinical observation and imaging methods (CT, ultrasound).

When symptoms of hemodynamic instability and/or peritonitis are recognized, emergency surgery should be performed under the right conditions.

Author details

Emrah Şahin[1*], İlhan Bali[2], Muhammed Said Dalkiliç[3], Mehmet Gençtürk[4], Merih Yilmaz[4], Burhan Hakan Kanat[5] and Selim Sözen[6]

1 Department of General Surgery, Doğanşehir Şehit Esra Köse Başaran State Hospital, Malatya, Turkey

2 Department of General Surgery, Namık Kemal University, Medical School, Tekirdağ, Turkey

3 Department of General Surgery, Marmara University, Medical School, Istanbul, Turkey

4 Department of General Surgery, Dr. HE Obesity Clinic, Kurtköy Ersoy Hospital, Istanbul, Turkey

5 Department of General Surgery, Turgut Özal University, Medical School, Malatya, Turkcy

6 Department of General Surgery, Sözen Surgery Clinic, Tekirdağ, Turkey

*Address all correspondence to: dr.emrahsahin@gmail.com

References

[1] Gad MA, Saber A, Farrag S, Shams ME, Ellabban GM. Incidence, patterns, and factors predicting mortality of abdominal injuries in trauma patients. North American Journal of Medical Sciences. 2012;**4**:129-134

[2] Sarsılmaz A, Kocakoç E. Abdominal Travma. Trd Sem. 2016;**4**:299-312

[3] Chalya PL, Mabula JB. Abdominal trauma experience over a two-year period at a tertiary hospital in north-western Tanzania: A prospective review of 396 cases. Tanzania Journal of Health Research. Oct 2013;**15**(4):230-239. PMID: 26591698

[4] Idriss AM, Tfeil Y, Baba JS, Boukhary SM, Hamad B, Abdllatif M, et al. Abdominal Trauma: Five Years Experience in National Centre Hospital, Mauritania. 2018

[5] Hardcastle TC, Finlayson M, van Heerden M, Johnson B, Samuel C, Muckart DJJ. The prehospital burden of disease due to trauma in KwaZulu-Natal: The need for Afrocentric trauma systems. World Journal of Surgery. 2013;**37**(7):1513-1525

[6] Hardcastle TC, Oosthuizen G, Clarke D, Lutge E. Trauma, a preventable burden of disease in South Africa: Review of the evidence, with a focus on KwaZulu-Natal. South African Health Review. 2016;**2016**(1):179-189

[7] Göksel K. Trakeobronşiyal Yaralanmalar. In: Ertekin C, Taviloğlu K, Güloğlu R, Kurtoğlu M, editors. Travma. 1. baskı. İstanbul: İstanbul Medikal Yayıncılık Ltd. Şti; 2005. pp. 841-845

[8] Soreide K. Epidemiology of major trauma. The British Journal of Surgery. 2009;**96**:697-698

[9] Wiewióra M, Sosada K, Piecuch J, Zurawiński W. The role of laparoscopy in abdominal trauma—Review of the literature. Wideochir Inne Tech Malo Inwazyjne. 2011;**6**:121-126

[10] Abdominal Trauma—Procedures—Clinical Pain Advisor [Internet]. 2022. Available from: https://www.clinicalpainadvisor.com/decision-support-in-medicine/anesthesiology/abdominal-trauma-procedures/

[11] John AM. In: Isenhour JL, Marx JA, editors. Abdominal Trauma. 7th ed. Missouri USA: Mosby, Inc; 2009. pp. 414-436

[12] Feliciano DV, Burch JM, Spjut-Patrinely V, Mattox KL, Jordan GL Jr. Abdominal gunshot wounds. An urban trauma center's experience with 300 consecutive patients. Annals of Surgery. 1988;**208**:362-370

[13] Rignault DP. Abdominal trauma in war. World Journal of Surgery. 1992;**16**:940-946

[14] Cushing BM, Clark DE, Cobean R, Schenarts PJ, Rutstein LA. Blunt and penetrating trauma—Has anything changed? The Surgical Clinics of North America. 1997;**77**(6):1321-1332

[15] Howes N, Walker T, Allorto NL, Oosthuizen GV, Clarke DL. Laparotomy for blunt abdominal trauma in a civilian trauma service. South African Journal of Surgery. 2012;**50**(2):30-32

[16] Bhagvan S, Turai M, Holden A, Ng A, Civil I. Predicting hollow viscus injury in blunt abdominal trauma with computed tomography. World Journal of Surgery. 2013;**37**(1):123-126

[17] Nagy KK, Roberts RR, Joseph KT, Smith RF, An GC, Bokhari F, et al. Experience with over 2500 diagnostic peritoneal lavages. Injury. 2000;**31**:479-482

[18] Davis RA, Shayne JP, Max MH, Woolfitt RA, Schwab W. The use of computerized axial tomography versus peritoneal lavage in the evaluation of blunt abdominal trauma: A prospective study. Surgery. 1985;**98**:845-850

[19] Mnguni MN, Muckart DJJ, Madiba TE. Abdominal trauma in Durban, South Africa: Factors influencing outcome. International Surgery. 2012;**97**(2):161-168

[20] Nicolau AE. Is laparoscopy still needed in blunt abdominal trauma. Chirurgia. 2011;**106**(1):59-66

[21] Tekin A, Küçükkartallar T, Vatansev C, Aksoy F, Belviranlı M, Kartal A. İntraabdominal Sepsiste Bogota Bag Uygulaması. Harran Üniversitesi Tıp Fakültesi Dergisi. 2006;**3**(3):77-81

[22] Suthar KD, Mewada BN. Abdominal injuries: An experience of 87 cases. The Journal of International Medical Research. 2012;**1**:1-8

[23] Mohamed El WA, Mohamed HR, Ali AN. Role of CT in Evaluation of Blunt Abdominal Trauma. International Journal of Medical Imaging. September 2015;**3**(5):89-93. DOI: 10.11648/j.ijmi.20150305.11

[24] Parks NA, Davis JW, Forman D, Lemaster D. Observation for nonoperative management of blunt liver injuries: How long is long enough? Journal of Trauma and Acute Care Surgery. 2011;**70**(3):626-629

[25] Caruso DM, Battistella FD, Owings JT, Lee SL, Samaco RC. Perihepatic packing of major liver injuries: Complications and mortality. Archives of Surgery. 1999;**134**(9): 958-962. discussion 962-963. DOI: 10.1001/archsurg.134.9.958

[26] Bruce PJP, Helmer SD, Harrison PB, Sirico T, Haan JM. Nonsurgical management of blunt splenic injury: Is it cost effective? American Journal of Surgery. 2011;**202**(6):810-816

[27] Skattum J, Titze TL, Dormagen JB, Aaberge IS, Bechensteen AG, Gaarder PI, et al. Preserved splenic function after angioembolisation of high grade injury. Injury. 2012;**43**(1):62-66

[28] Ntundu SH, Herman AM, Kishe A, Babu H, Jahanpour OF, Msuya D, et al. Patterns and outcomes of patients with abdominal trauma on operative management from northern Tanzania: A prospective single Centre observational study. BMC Surgery. 2019;**19**(1):1-10. DOI: 10.1186/s12893-019-0530-8

[29] Okuş A, Sevinç B, Ay S, Arslan K, Karahan Ö, Eryılmaz MA. Conservative management of abdominal injuries. Turkish Journal of Surgery/Ulusal cerrahi Derg. 2013;**29**(4):153

Chapter 2

Appropriate Protective Measures for the Prevention of Animal-related Goring Injuries

Ashok Kumar Puranik and Althea Vency Cardoz

Abstract

The most common cause of morbidity and mortality worldwide in the age group of 10–49 years is road traffic accidents. Other than road traffic accidents multiple other factors add to the burden of injuries which include self-harm, occupational hazards, animal attack injuries and industrial accidents. Animal attack injuries are seen all over the world. Other than a few case reports and case series, this mode of injury is highly under-reported. Hence, the global burden of this disease is unknown. Due to the rapid deforestation, the number of animal attack injuries is increasing. These injuries can be caused by wild as well as domesticated animals. The attack can be due to a direct encounter with an animal or due to road traffic accident. Bulls are ferocious animals that are used for sporting events. They are also used for farming and livestock rearing. Injuries caused by bulls can be due to direct attacks by an unprovoked animal, road traffic accidents, or sporting events. The penetrating injury caused by the bull horn has its characteristic pattern. Treatment of bull horn injuries requires a multidisciplinary team. Creating awareness and enforcing laws can help in preventing such injuries.

Keywords: animal attack injuries, goring injuries, bull horn injuries, bull gore, penetrating injuries

1. Introduction

Injury is the leading cause of morbidity and mortality all over the world. The most common cause responsible for global DALYs is road traffic accidents. Road traffic accidents were responsible for 6.6% and 5.9% of global DALY's in the age group of 10–24 years and 25–49 years respectively in 2019 [1]. Animal-related injuries are commonly seen all over the world. Attacks by wild animals as well as domesticated animals are commonly seen. These injuries are highly under-reported with only a few case series and case reports being published. They add a significant number to global mortality and morbidity and are a cause of concern in today's world. These animals cause injuries by directly attacking humans or by causing road traffic accidents.

Bull horn injuries are common in different parts of the world where farming and livestock rearing is practised as well as in places where bulls are used for sports events. Bull horns can cause blunt, penetrating or mixed injuries. The injuries are most

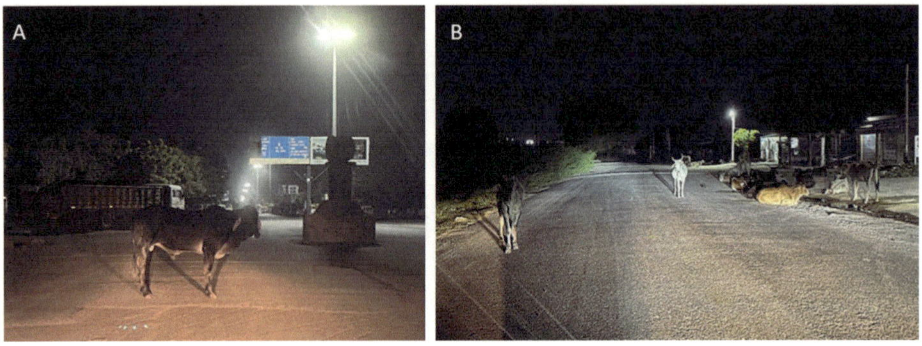

Figure 1.
A and B. Image showing Indian bulls on the street which are a potential cause of road traffic accidents.

commonly seen over the abdomen and perineal region though injuries can be present anywhere from the head to toe. In low- or middle-income countries (LMIC), stray cattle, as well as domesticated cattle, are seen on the streets which can lead to road traffic accidents causing multiple injuries.

The injuries caused by penetrating bull horns have their characteristics such as multiple paths of injuries, a large area of tissue damage, creation of cavities, twists and inoculation of anaerobic and aerobic bacteria. There are four types of bull horn wounds. They are (i) sideway thrust caused due to tangential injury causing contusions, (ii) jab wounds where the tip of the horn causes injury, (iii) misleading injury where the entry point is away from the site of deep injury and (iv) goring injury in which there is a deep wound that penetrates the fascia and muscle [2].

Prevention of injuries due to bull horns can help in decreasing morbidity and mortality. Appropriate laws need to be enforced regarding bullfighting. In India, stray cattle and bulls need to be taken off the highways and kept in appropriate infrastructure where they can be taken care of (**Figure 1**).

2. Mechanism and patterns of injury

Injury caused by bull goring is complex and hence it is necessary to know the mechanism behind these injuries. The bull initially lowers his head by neck flexion while charging toward the subject. After engaging, it extends its neck driving one or both horns into the subject. The weight along with the acceleration of the bull causes the generation of a tremendous force at the site of entry. The bull then tosses his head in a circular motion causing a shearing injury. Due to the flexion of the neck during charging, the most common primary site of injury is the abdomen, perineum and upper thigh. During bullfighting the individual faces the bull, hence the injuries are situated anteriorly while during running the injuries are found posteriorly [3].

Secondary injuries are caused due throwing, stomping or trampling and secondary penetrating injuries. Throwing can result in blunt trauma due to impact on the ground or the surroundings. This can cause intra-cranial injuries, spinal injuries, thoracoabdominal injuries and fractures. Stomping can cause acute life-threatening injuries. Factors determining the severity of the injury depend on the velocity and weight of the bull. Trampling occurs while running causing additional injury by multiple bulls. Secondary penetrating injuries occur if an individual attempts to stand after being thrown and the bull focuses on him as a target. The bull charges toward the individual causing secondary goring injuries. These injuries are located on the upper body as the individual is usually in a kneeling down position [3]. This causes penetrating injuries to the head, face, neck or thorax.

Injuries by bulls can also occur due to motor vehicular accidents. In LMIC like in India, cattle wander in the streets which can lead to motor vehicle crashes causing a wide spectrum of injuries. In areas where bulls are used for farming and livestock rearing, unprovoked injuries occur while handling and taking care of the livestock, this can lead to penetrating or blunt injuries.

3. Organ specific injuries

Injuries due to bull horns can affect any part of the human body. A retrospective study from January 2002 to March 2016 of penetrating bull horn injuries published from Maharashtra, India reported 67 cases. The most common site of injury was the abdomen. This was followed by the perineum, back and lower limbs. The least commonly affected site was the head and neck. The lower part of the abdomen was more commonly affected as compared to the rest of the abdomen [2]. Another retrospective study carried out from January 1978 to December 2019 in Spain reported a total of 572 cases of bull horn injury. The most frequent site of injury was the lower extremity, perineum and abdomen. The most commonly injured intra-abdominal organ was the intestine and liver. Their study reported an overall mortality of 0.87% [4]. A prospective study from June 2017 to March 2019 conducted in Tamil Nadu, India reported 42 cases. The most common site of injury was the trunk (55%) followed by the perineum (19%). The most common mechanism was penetrating injury (59.5%). Blunt injuries were seen in 31% of the patients while 9.5% of patients had both blunt and penetrating injuries. In abdominal injuries, liver injury was seen in three patients, splenic injury in one patient, renal injury in one patient and three patients had bowel perforation [5].

3.1 Head, face and neck

The incidence of head injuries as reported in a study in India was 1.6% [5]. Injuries due to bull can cause blunt or penetrating head injuries. Blunt injuries can cause fractures of the scalp bones as well as intracranial hematomas such as extradural hematoma, subdural hematoma, subarachnoid hematoma and intraparenchymal hematoma. A case of penetrating head injury with retained horn within the brain in a 3-year-old child was reported in India [6]. Individuals present with a history of loss of consciousness and/or with a low GCS.

Face can be involved due to penetrating or blunt injuries. Blunt injuries can result in fractures of facial bones and contusions over the face. Penetrating neck injury is defined as any injury that extends deep to the platysma. It can cause injury to major vessels, esophagus and the trachea. Patients can present with an unsecured airway and in shock. Injuries involving zone 1 and 2 of the neck require immediate exploration. A case of traumatic tooth intrusion in a six-year-old boy was reported in India. It was managed by extraction of intruded teeth to prevent interference with the eruption of permanent teeth [7]. A case of cervical esophageal perforation following a penetrating bull gore injury to the neck was reported from India. The patient was managed surgically with a primary repair over a T-tube and a feeding jejunostomy [8]. A case of complete tracheal transection following penetrating bull horn injury was reported from India. The patient was managed by emergency surgery. Since the distal tracheal end had retracted into the mediastinum, the patient was induced for surgery using percutaneous femoro-femoral cardiopulmonary bypass [9]. A case of penetrating bull horn injury to the neck causing mandible fracture and injury to the branches of facial vessels was reported from Mexico. The patient underwent emergency surgery during which the mandible fracture was fixed using plates and screws and the branches of facial vessels were ligated [10].

3.2 Torso injuries

Penetrating injury to the abdomen is commonly seen as injury to the lower abdomen. It can cause injuries to the bowel, urinary bladder, major vessels of the abdomen and solid organs like the liver, spleen, and kidneys. It can also cause evisceration of the bowel or omentum. Penetrating abdominal injuries can also extend to the thorax after injuring the diaphragm. Diaphragmatic injuries can have delayed presentation. Abdominal injuries can also occur due to blunt trauma due to secondary mechanisms. Blunt injury can cause solid organ injuries, abdominal wall hernias, mesenteric injuries and bowel injuries. A case of traumatic abdominal wall hernia following blunt abdominal trauma due to bull horn which was repaired by open mesh hernioplasty using a 15 × 15 cm polypropylene mesh was reported from India [11]. Another case of traumatic direct inguinal hernia following blunt bull horn injuries was reported from India [12]. A delayed presentation of intercostodiaphragmatic hernia following a forgotten penetrating injury was reported from India [13]. A case of penetrating abdominal injury causing terminal ileal perforation was reported from India. The patient was managed surgically by resection of the involved segment and ileoascending anastomosis [2].

Injuries to the thorax can be due to blunt or penetrating trauma. Penetrating trauma can cause open pneumothorax. The horn can penetrate the thorax and cause

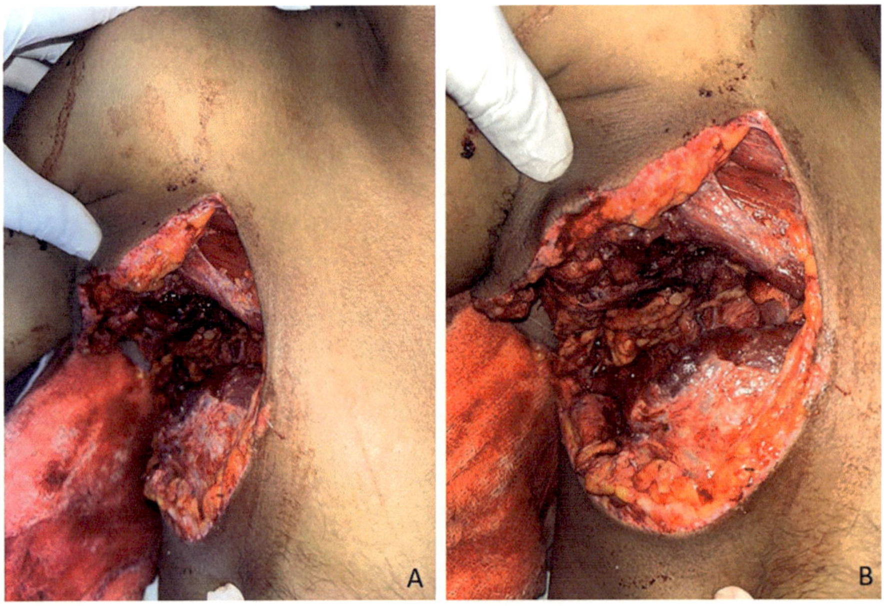

Figure 2.
A and B. Image showing penetrating bull horn injury to the right hemithorax.

injuries to the lungs, bronchus, heart, and major vessels. Blunt trauma can cause rib fractures which can result in hemothorax, pneumothorax, and lung contusions. Injuries to major vessels can cause massive hemothorax which can be life-threatening. Penetrating injuries to the heart can be life-threatening. A case of blunt thoracic injury due to being hit by a domestic bull resulting in right-sided rib fractures with flail segment and hemothorax was reported in India. The patient was managed with an intercostal tube drainage system and epidural anesthesia (see **Figure 2**) [14].

3.3 Perineal injuries

The perineum is one of the common sites of injury due to a penetrating bull horn. The perineal wound may be superficial or extend deeper to involve the pelvic organs. Perineal trauma can involve the anal canal, perineal body, urethra, vagina in females, scrotum and testis in males and pelvic organs like urinary bladder, reproductive organs and the rectum. Injuries can also involve the intra-abdominal organs. Patients with a perineal injury can present with bleeding per vagina, bleeding per-rectum, prolapse of pelvic organs, bowel injury, and injury to major vessels causing hypotensive shock. The delayed presentation can be in the form of a recto-vaginal fistula or a recto-urethral fistula. A case of traumatic urethrorectal fistula due to bull horn injury was reported from India. It was initially managed by diversion sigmoid colostomy and suprapubic cystostomy [15]. Two cases of goring injury to the vagina were reported from India. Both cases were managed operatively after initial resuscitation [16]. A case of penetrating bull gore injury to the perineum with urinary bladder perforation and pneumoperitoneum which was managed surgically was reported from India (**Figure 3**) [17].

3.4 Extremities

Lower extremities are more commonly involved than upper extremities. Bull goring can result in lacerations which can be simple or there can be extensive tissue loss, fractures involving long bones and injuries to major vessels of the limb. These wounds are highly contaminated with vegetative matter, pieces of clothing, soil and microorganisms such as anaerobes, gram-positive, gram-negative bacteria and fungi. They also have a high risk of transmitting tetanus.

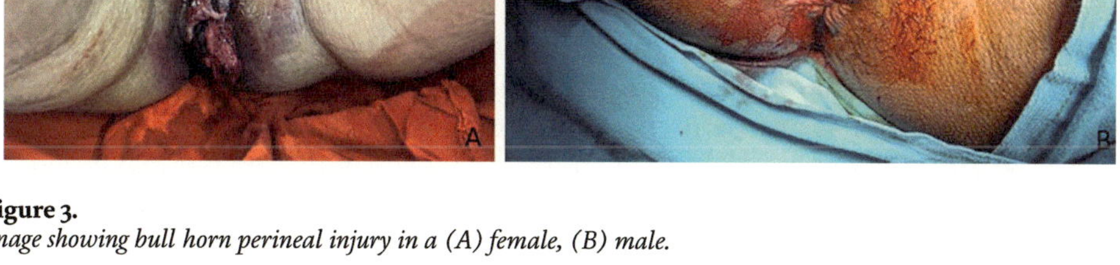

Figure 3.
Image showing bull horn perineal injury in a (A) female, (B) male.

3.5 Vascular injuries

Vascular injuries are seen during penetrating injury to the extremities, head and neck region, abdomen, thorax, perineum, back and lumbar region. A case of external iliac artery thrombosis which was repaired using the endovascular technique was reported from Spain [18].

4. Management

Patients usually present with multiple injuries following an attack by bulls. Management of an individual with bull goring injuries requires teamwork. Adequate pre-hospital care should be provided during the transportation of the patient to the hospital. Following ATLS protocols, the patient is managed primarily by maintaining Airway and stabilization of the cervical spine, breathing, circulation, neurological evaluation and control of exposure and environment. Continuous monitoring is done using an ECG, pulse oximeter and blood pressure monitors. Urinary and gastric catheters can be placed in patients with multiple injuries. A chest X-ray, pelvic X-ray and an eFAST are done as adjuncts to the primary survey. Patients with open wounds need to be vaccinated against tetanus. Once the patient is stabilized, a secondary survey is done to look for the extent of injuries. Based on the injuries a computed tomography (CT) of the head, chest, abdomen, contrast urography or angiography can be done. Penetrating injuries will require exploration under anesthesia after initial stabilization and evaluation of the patient. These individuals have to be started on triple antibiotics due to the dirty nature of the wound. Careful exploration and evaluation of the entire trajectory of the wound and removal of foreign material are necessary.

Individuals presenting with unstable vitals need to be resuscitated initially with intravenous fluids, tranexamic acid 1gm and a requisition for blood for crossmatching should be sent. If the patients are non-responders to initial resuscitation, they have to be shifted to the operating room. The source of bleeding in these patients needs to be identified and controlled. Such patients require damage control surgery as prolonged surgery in them can be fatal. The goals of damage control surgery are to stop any active bleeding and control of contamination. The minimal required amount of surgery required to stabilize the patient is done so that the patient physiological status can be corrected. Further resuscitation is then continued in the intensive care unit. Definitive surgery is carried out within 24–72 h after stabilization of the patient in the intensive care unit.

Penetrating injuries to the abdomen may present with hemodynamic instability, herniation of intraabdominal contents or with hemodynamically stable vitals. Patients with evisceration require exploration in the operating room after initial resuscitation. Unstable patients may require a laparotomy. In stable patients with penetrating injury who require exploration, a diagnostic laparoscopy can be considered. This can prevent the morbidity of an exploratory laparotomy. On exploration, patients may have an injury to the bowel, urinary bladder or solid organs. Bowel injuries may require primary repair, resection of the involved segment with anastomosis or creation of a stoma in patients requiring damage control surgery. Colonic injuries may require a protective diversion ileostomy after primary repair of the injury site. Urinary bladder injury can be repaired primarily by taking care not to injure the ureteric openings in the bladder. Suprapubic cystostomy can be done for drainage of urine and to allow healing of the urinary bladder. Injury to the liver can be managed by packing, pressure or Pringle maneuver. Grade four or five splenic injury or splenic injury with active bleeding may require splenectomy. Injury to major intra-abdominal vessels should be repaired primarily or with a graft. Blunt injuries to the abdomen with hemodynamically stable vitals can be managed conservatively with continuous monitoring in an intensive care unit and the presence of a twenty-four-hour availability of an operating room. Blunt injuries with features of peritonitis may require exploration. The presence of diaphragmatic injuries needs to be evaluated during exploration. If any diaphragmatic injury is identified, it can be primarily repaired. A randomized controlled study published in India on the management of penetrating injuries concluded that patients with penetrating injury to the anterior abdominal wall with hemodynamically stable vitals can be managed by serial observation after obtaining a CECT and in the absence of injuries requiring immediate surgery as compared to diagnostic laparoscopy in a centre that has 24-hour availability of operating room facilities, radiology facilities and an intensive care unit. This reduced the rate of non-therapeutic surgeries [19]. The presence of retroperitoneal injuries need to be identified during laparotomy. Injuries involving zone 1 of the retroperitoneum need to be explored after obtaining proximal and distal vascular control. Hematomas in zone 2 and 3 need to be explored only if they are pulsatile or expanding. If the tract of penetrating injury is extending to the retroperitoneum then the area has to be explored to look for injuries [20].

Penetrating injuries to the perineum require exploration after initial resuscitation. The wound needs to be evaluated for the extent of injury and organs involved. Patients with perineal penetrating bull horn injury may present with features of peritonitis and may require exploratory laparotomy along with local wound exploration. The perineal wound needs to be evaluated for communication with the urinary bladder, urethra, rectum and anal canal, vagina in females and scrotum and testis in males. The superficial injury needs to be closed in layers. Injuries involving the rectum and anal canal need to be repaired. A diversion sigmoid colostomy may be created to allow for healing of the wound. Injuries involving the vagina need to be repaired in layers. Precaution has to be taken while repairing the posterior wall of the vagina and anterior wall of rectum to avoid the formation of rectovaginal fistula and between anterior wall of vagina and urethra or urinary bladder to prevent the formation of fistula in females. In males, precaution needs to be taken to avoid the formation of the recto-urethral fistula or a fistula between the rectum and urinary bladder. Large perineal wounds involving the anal sphincter may require the creation of diversion sigmoid colostomy to prevent soiling of wounds. Concomitant intra-abdominal injuries need to be evaluated and appropriately managed. Perineal wounds with loss of tissue require initial debridement and wound management followed by delayed closure primarily with a reconstruction.

Patients with immediate life-threatening thoracic injuries should be identified and managed during the primary survey. These include airway obstruction, tension pneumothorax, pericardial tamponade, open pneumothorax, massive hemothorax and flail chest. The potentially life-threatening thoracic injuries are aortic injuries, tracheobronchial injuries, myocardial contusion, pulmonary contusion, diaphragmatic injuries and esophageal injuries. These injuries need to be identified during a secondary survey as these injuries have subtle signs and can be easily missed if a high index of suspicion is not maintained to look for these injuries. Emergency room thoracotomy is indicated in individuals who have a penetrating cardiac injury and have received cardio-pulmonary resuscitation for less than 15 minutes. The aim of an emergency room thoracotomy is control of hemorrhage, open cardiac massage, cardiac tamponade release, cross-clamping of descending thoracic aorta to cut off arterial supply to the distal body and preserve blood supply to the heart and brain in major penetrating injury to the abdomen, repair of cardiac or pulmonary injury and prevention of air embolism. Emergency thoracotomy is indicated in massive hemothorax which is defined as more than 1500 ml of blood in one hemithorax or when 150–200 ml of blood drains per hour for the next 2–4 h in an ICD bag and persistent hemodynamic instability in the presence of ongoing transfusion. In an open pneumothorax injury, an ICD needs to be placed after creating a flap valve over the wound. After the initial stabilization of the patient, the wound needs to be explored in an operation theater. The margins are debrided as they are heavily contaminated and the wound is closed in layers. The majority of thoracic injuries can be managed by placement of an intercostal tube drain. The ICD can be removed within 2–3 days after obtaining full lung expansion and minimal output from the drain. Patients with residual hemothorax that does not drain with an intercostal tube drain can be considered for VATS drainage. Patients with flail chest with respiratory compromise may require ventilatory support or rib fixation. Esophageal injuries presenting within 24 h can be managed surgically by primary repair. A feeding jejunostomy may be created to allow for postoperative enteral feeding. Delayed presentation of esophageal injury needs to be evaluated. In case of mediastinitis with septic shock, the patient needs surgical management. In cases of contained perforation, conservative management can be tried, if the patient deteriorates on conservative management, then the patient can be taken for surgery. Adequate analgesic support should be provided in the form of epidural analgesia or erector spinae blocks and intravenous analgesics. Chest physiotherapy and respirometry are necessary to prevent post-traumatic pneumonia and for early recovery.

Penetrating wounds to the extremity need to be explored after initial resuscitation. A CT angiography may be needed to evaluate for the presence of vascular injury. Superficial wounds may be closed primarily after debridement of devitalized tissue. Wounds with tissue loss may require serial debridement, regular dressing, and use of a vacuum-assisted closure dressing followed by delayed closure. Delayed closure may require tissue reconstruction using skin grafts, rotational flaps or free flaps. Vascular injuries need to be repaired if presented within 6 h of injury. Primary repair of the injured vessel may be done. In case of tissue loss, a reverse saphenous graft may be placed. Delayed presentation of more than 6 h may cause ischemia of the limb which may require amputation.

Penetrating neck injuries need to be evaluated in the operating room. Injuries involving the trachea need an emergency tracheostomy done in the emergency room to maintain the airway. A CT angiography needs to be done if the patient is hemodynamically stable to look for the extent of injury and presence of any vascular injury. Hemodynamically unstable patients need to be taken to the operating room after maintaining the airway. The wound needs to be evaluated to identify injuries to major structures. Tracheal injuries need to be repaired. A tracheostomy may be needed in injuries with tissue loss. Injury to major vessels can be primarily repaired. Cervical esophageal injury may be repaired primarily or an esophagostomy can be created. A feeding jejunostomy may be required to allow for enteral feeding in the postoperative period. Injury to soft tissue can be debrided to remove the devitalized tissue and closed in layers. Injuries involving the thyroid gland or salivary glands may require partial or complete excision depending on the extent of the injury.

Majority of injuries to the head can be managed conservatively in the intensive care unit. Penetrating injury to the head requires surgery after initial resuscitation. Blunt injuries causing intracranial bleed requiring surgery are hemorrhage causing

DOI: http://dx.doi.org/10.5772/intechopen.108438

midline shift, raised intracranial pressure, extradural hemorrhage, infratentorial bleed, and open depressed fracture of the cranial vault. A decompressive craniotomy is done. Depressed fracture is treated by elevation of fracture segment and debridement of the wound. Since bull horn penetrating injuries are contaminated wounds, a prosthesis is avoided during primary surgery.

Management of bull horn injuries requires a multidisciplinary team. A holistic approach toward patient care is necessary for a positive outcome for the patients. Patients with polytrauma need to be referred to a higher centre with acute care facilities or a trauma centre as soon as possible for a better outcome of the patient.

5. Conclusion

Bull horn injuries are commonly seen in rural India as they are used for domestic and farming purposes. It is also commonly seen in Spain where traditional bullfighting is a sport. Bull horn injuries have special features that make them unique as compared to other modes of injuries. Injuries due to bull horns can vary from penetrating injury to blunt injury to both. Management of bull horn injury requires a holistic approach by a multidisciplinary team. Early referral to a tertiary care centre is necessary for the survival of the patient. Injuries caused due to bulls are a preventable mechanism. The three E's of trauma prevention should be followed which are engineering, education and enforcement. Creating awareness among the people in places where bullfighting is a sport such as Spain, Latin America and certain parts of India about the severity of injuries caused due to bullfighting can help in preventing injuries during these sports events. Appropriate protective measures should be undertaken and rules regarding the same should be enforced by the government to prevent injuries caused during these sporting events. Any individual not following such rules and regulations should be penalized. Building infrastructure to take care of stray animals, appropriate fighting grounds to prevent injuries during sporting events, use of protective equipment, and availability of a medical team on-site to attend to the individuals and take care of life-threatening conditions should be enforced by the government. Appropriate rules and regulations should be enforced by the government to prevent the presence of stray cattle and bulls on the Indian streets. This can prevent a significant number of road traffic accidents caused by bulls thus decreasing the burden of disease.

Acknowledgement

Usually, the acknowledgements section includes the names of people or institutions who in some way contributed to the work, but do not fit the criteria to be listed as the authors.

The authorship criteria are listed in our Authorship Policy: https://www.intechopen.com/page/authorship-policy.

This section of your manuscript may also include funding information.

Conflict of interest

The authors declare no conflict of interest.

Notes/thanks/other declarations

Place any other declarations, such as "Notes", "Thanks", etc. in before the References section. Assign the appropriate heading. Do NOT put your short biography in this section. It will be removed.

Author details

Ashok Kumar Puranik[1*] and Althea Vency Cardoz[2]

1 All India Institute of Medical Sciences, Guwahati, India

2 All India Institute of Medical Sciences, Jodhpur, India

*Address all correspondence to: puranik_6@hotmail.com

References

[1] Vos T, Lim SS, Abbafati C, Abbas KM, Abbasi M, Abbasifard M, et al. Global burden of 369 diseases and injuries in 204 countries and territories, 1990-2019: A systematic analysis for the global burden of disease study 2019. The Lancet. 17 Oct 2020;**396**(10258):1204-1222

[2] Gajbhiye AS, Shamkuwar A, Bokade A, Nasare V, Jehughale K, Agrawal A. Surgical management of bull horn injury. International Surgery Journal. 2016;**3**(4):2041-2045

[3] Spiotta AM, Matoses SM. Neurosurgical considerations after bull goring during festivities in Spain and Latin America. Neurosurgery. 2011;**69**(2):455-461

[4] Hernández AM, Ramos DM, Moreno MVG, Mohamed NA, Loscos EL, Hilario EA, et al. Bull horn injuries. A 40-year retrospective study with 572 patients. The American Journal of Surgery. 2021;**222**(2):446-452

[5] Nagarajan S, Jena NN, Davey K, Douglas K, Smith J, Blanchard J. Patients presenting with bull-related injuries to a southern Indian emergency department. The Western Journal of Emergency Medicine. 2020;**21**(6):291-294

[6] Kumar P, Kulshreshtha V, Kumar A, Jaiswal G, Gupta TK. Bull horn head injury with retained horn in brain: A rare case report. Journal of Pediatric Neurosciences. 2018;**13**(2):229-233

[7] Bhoil R, Bramta M, Bhoil R. Bull horn injury causing traumatic tooth intrusion—Ultrasound and CT imaging. African Journal of Emergency Medicine. 2020;**10**(2):99-102

[8] Vaddavalli VV, Singh C, Abuji K, Kaman L, Savlania A. A bull gore penetrating injury to the neck presenting with esophageal perforation: A case report. Cureus. 28 Mar 2022;**14**(3)

[9] Parage F, Vashisht A, Sisodia V, Sanyal A, Singh S, Kamal K, et al. Reconstruction of complete tracheal transection with cardiopulmonary bypass support following bull horn injury in neck during coronavirus disease 19 pandemic lockdown. Indian Journal of Thoracic and Cardiovascular Surgery. 2021;**37**(4):442-446

[10] Luis FG. Bull horn injure in neck and face bones: Case report and literature review. Corpus. 2019;**2**(4):3

[11] Bodda AK, Sasmal PK, Mishra S, Shettar A. Mesh hernioplasty in emergency repair of traumatic abdominal wall hernia following bull horn injury. BML Case Reports. 2021;**14**(7):e244384

[12] Chate N, Deshmukh S, Dange A. Inguinal hernia resulting from bull horn injury: Letters to the editor. ANZ Journal of Surgery. 2011;**81**(12):943-943

[13] Nabi G, Seenu V, Misra MC. Intercostodiaphragmatic hernia secondary to a bull gore injury: A delayed detection. The Indian Journal of Chest Diseases & Allied Sciences. 2002;**44**(3):187-189

[14] Bull horn injury to chest–Management and review of literature. Journal of Anesthesia and Critical Care: Open Access [Internet]. 2017;8(3). Available from: https://medcraveonline.com/JACCOA/JACCOA-08-00305.pdf

[15] Pal DK, Bora V, Bisoi SC, Dwivedi US. Urethrorectal fistula by bull horn injury. Journal of the Indian Medical Association. 2002;**100**(1):47

[16] Kulkarni MR, Gangadharaiah M, Kulkarni SR. Bull gore injury of the vagina. Journal of Clinical and Diagnostic Research. 2013;7(1):158-159

[17] Santhosh R, Barad AK, Ghalige HS, Sridartha K, Sharma MB. Perineal bull gore with urinary bladder perforation and pneumoperitoneum. Journal of Clinical and Diagnostic Research. 2013;7(5):902-904

[18] Maldonado-Fernández N, Martínez-Gámez FJ, Mata-Campos JE, Galán-Zafra M, Sánchez-Maestre ML. Bull horn injuries: Endovascular repair of an external iliac artery thrombosis. Cirugía Española. 2013;**91**(5):340-342

[19] Kaur S, Bagaria D, Kumar A, Priyadarshini P, Choudhary N, Sagar S, et al. Contrast-enhanced computed tomography abdomen versus diagnostic laparoscopy-based management in patients with penetrating abdominal trauma: A randomised controlled trial. European Journal of Trauma and Emergency Surgery. 18 Aug 2022:1-10

[20] Williams NS, O'Connell PR, McCaskie AW, editors. Bailey and Love's Short Practice of Surgery. 27th ed. Boca Raton, FL: CRC Press; 2017

Chapter 3

Management of Duodenal Injuries

José Miguel Aceves-Ayala, David Jacob Álvarez-Chávez, Clara Elizabeth Valdez-Cruz, Cristhian Felipe Montoya-Salazar, Carlos Alfredo Bautista-López, Cesar Alberto Ortiz-Orozco, Wence Francisco Villalvazo-Zuñiga and Pablo Francisco Rojas-Solís

Abstract

The duodenum is mostly a retroperitoneal structure, composed by 4 segments (D1-D4) and surrounded by other vital organs like pancreas or great vessels. Injuries to this organ are rare and difficult to diagnose, with an incidence of 1–5% in cases of abdominal trauma. The most common causes of duodenal injuries are gunshot wounds and stabbing. Duodenal injuries are often associated with other organ injuries, thus delaying diagnosis in some cases and increasing the risk of complications. When diagnosed at optimum timing, it can be treated with relatively low mortality rates. Great number of repair techniques exist and the treatment of choice depends on the surgeon's experience and hemodynamic stability of the patient, with the goal of preserving life and preventing a major complication such as leak or fistula. Outcomes are good, and the prognosis is tightly ligated to associated injuries, thus high index of suspicion and applying ATLS and surgery trauma principles are essential.

Keywords: hollow viscus, blunt trauma, anastomosis, pyloric exclusion, acute care surgery

1. Introduction

Duodenal injuries are rare and difficult to diagnose [1], with a reported incidence of 1–5% in cases of abdominal trauma [2, 3]. In a review by García-Santos et al., where 23 case series of duodenal injury were included, the ratio of penetrating and blunt abdominal trauma was found to be 3.9: 1. Among the penetrating injuries, 81% were caused by gunshot wounds and 19% by stabbing [2]. Among blunt abdominal trauma cases, the most frequent mechanism was motor vehicle accidents in 85% [2] due to crushing of the duodenum between the steering wheel and the spine [4].

In general, it is estimated that 4.3% of patients with a history of duodenal trauma present intra-abdominal lesions at the duodenal level; in various case series they range from 3–7%, reporting a male–female ratio of 5:1 with an age disposition of 16 to 30 years in 70% of the cases.

Mortality associated with this type of injury ranges from 18 to 30% [1, 2]. Early deaths are caused by massive hemorrhage from major vascular injuries or associated traumatic brain injuries, while late deaths are associated with sepsis, duodenal fistulae, and multi-organ failure. It is imperative to recognize these lesions in a timely manner, since the most important risk factor associated with mortality is the delay between diagnosis and treatment [2], since a delay in diagnosis in the first 24 hours can increase mortality up to 4 times. Other risk factors that increase the mortality rate include the presence of associated pancreatic injury and common bile duct injury.

Because the duodenum is surrounded by vital structures and organs, it presents associated intra-abdominal injuries in 68–100% [1, 2, 4]. The kinematics of trauma play an important role in the severity and injured organs; the abdominal structures with the highest rate of injury are: liver (17%), pancreas (12%), small intestine (11%), colon (13%), stomach (9%), bile duct (6%), kidney and urinary tract (6.5%), spleen (4.1%) and vascular injuries such as aorta, vena cava and porta up to 15%, the latter being the ones with the highest mortality due to the high possibility of massive hemorrhage [2].

With reference to the duodenum, an analysis of 1042 patients found that the most frequent site of injury was the second segment (36%), followed by the third portion (18%), and the fourth portion (15%). The least frequently injured portion of the duodenum was the first (13%), and in 18% of the cases, injuries to multiple portions were found [2].

2. Duodenal injuries

2.1 Surgical anatomy

The duodenum is the first portion of the small intestine, it has an approximate length of 30 cm. It is divided into four segments; the first segment has an approximate length of five centimeters, it crosses over the muscular ring of the pylorus towards the vesicular neck. The common bile duct, portal vein, inferior vena cava and the gastroduodenal artery are found behind it; anteriorly, it is related to the hepatic square lobe; superiorly, with the gastroepiploic foramen and inferiorly, with the pancreatic head. This segment is irrigated by the supraduodenal artery and the posterosuperior pancreaticoduodenal branch of the gastroduodenal artery, which is a branch of the common hepatic artery.

As of its second segment, it becomes retroperitoneal, with an average length of 7. 5 cm, referentially from the vesicular neck to the fourth lumbar vertebra; it is divided into two portions (supramesocolic and inframesocolic) since it is crossed by the transverse colon and the mesocolon. Due to its descending disposition, it crosses in front of the right kidney, right ureter, right renal vessels, psoas major and inferior vena cava. Its first half is retroperitoneal and it becomes intraperitoneal distally. The major duodenal papilla is located in the middle portion.

Its third segment has a length of 10 cm, it is located approximately five centimeters from the right side of the third or fourth lumbar vertebra, to the left side of the abdominal aorta, it has a transverse disposition in a leftward direction relating with the ureter, the right gonadal vessels, psoas muscle and the inferior vena cava, as well as with the uncinate process of the pancreas; the inferior pancreaticoduodenal artery is found in a groove located between the duodenum and the pancreas.

The fourth segment is ascending, has a length of 2.5 centimeters, has an oblique disposition in a cranial direction, and ends in the duodenojejunal junction, which is suspended by the ligament of Treitz, being found approximately 4 centimeters below and medial to the ninth costal cartilage. It is anteriorly related to the left sympathetic trunk, and its distal end approaches the terminal portion of the inferior mesenteric vein, the left ureter and the left kidney.

The last three segments of the duodenum receive their irrigation from an anterior and a posterior arcade, from which the pancreatic and duodenal branches arise [5].

2.2 Diagnosis

The diagnosis of duodenal injury is usually difficult, especially in cases of blunt trauma, since the symptoms may not be very obvious, however, it may present data of abdominal tenderness or peritonitis in the initial evaluation, highly suggestive of intra-abdominal injuries, but unspecific to a duodenal injury [4, 6].

FAST (Focused Assessment with Sonography in Trauma) is a widely accepted and useful method in cases of blunt abdominal trauma due to its ability to obtain faster results and with practically zero invasion. However, it has a low sensitivity for duodenal injuries, since up to 30% of patients with some type of retroperitoneal injury, including the duodenum, may present a FAST without alterations, determining the need to perform other extension studies such as abdominal computed tomography (CT) [4, 6].

Abdominal X-ray in standing position may suggest duodenal injury if right psoas muscle effacement or retroperitoneal air is found, however, it is unreliable [1, 2]. CT is one of the best methods to diagnose duodenal injuries in hemodynamically stable patients, even without the need to use water-soluble contrast [1]. The sensitivity of abdominal CT to detect biliopancreatic and duodenal (BPD) injuries approaches an 83%, decreasing to 79% for biliopancreatic (BP) injuries and 50% in bilioduodenal (BD) injuries [6, 7].

CT findings of duodenal injury include wall thickening, right pararenal or periduodenal fluid, decreased enhancement in the injured duodenal segment, and accumulation of clots near the injury site, visualized as a collection of heterogeneous fluid ("sign of the sentinel clot") [4]. Findings that are suggestive of duodenal perforation are the presence of air in the retroperitoneum, wall disruption and contrast extravasation [2, 6].

Magnetic resonance imaging (MRI) is more sensitive than CT for the detection of low-grade injuries, however, it is more expensive and lacks utility in the context of trauma, its use is generally reserved for the evaluation of associated pancreatic or biliary ductal injuries [6].

2.3 Classification

Different scales have been developed to classify the severity of duodenal injuries in the context of trauma, such as the World Society for Emergency Surgery (WSES) and the American Association for the Surgery of Trauma (AAST) classifications, the latter classifies duodenal injuries in 5 grades (**Table 1**) [8].

Instead, the WSES divides injury into four classes, considering the AAST classification and the hemodynamic status [9]:

I. Mild (AAST I)

II. Moderate (AAST II)

III. Severe (AAST III-V)

IV. Hemodynamic instability (AAST I-V of duodenal-biliary-pancreatic injury)

Grade	Type of injury	Description of injury
I	Hematoma Laceration	Involving single portion of duodenum Partial thickness, no perforation
II	Hematoma Laceration	Involving more than one portion Disruption <50% of circumference
III	Laceration	Disruption 50–75% circumference of D2 Disruption 50–100% circumference of D_1
IV	Laceration	Disruption >75% circumference of D_2 Involving ampulla or distal common bile duct
V	Laceration	Massive disruption of duodenopancreatic complex Devascularization of duodenum

Table 1.
AAST duodenal injury scale: D1, D2, D3, and D4 indicates the first, second, third and fourth segments of the duodenum, respectively (adapted from [8]).

This premise arises from the need to standardize local and regional anatomical disruptions, which allow determining the characteristics of the injury conditioned by the kinematics of the trauma; allowing the development of systematic approach strategies that have a positive impact on patient morbidity and mortality [9].

2.4 Management

The initial management is in accordance with the Advance Trauma Life Support (ATLS), hence, patients with hemodynamic instability, peritonitis or evisceration, must be transferred promptly to the operating room (OR). Hemodynamically stable patients with CT findings of low-grade injuries can be treated non-operatively.

2.4.1 Non-operative management (NOM)

Hemodynamically stable patients with CT findings of duodenal hematoma (AAST grade I-I) and no other associated injuries requiring surgical intervention are good candidates to conservative management [3]. The cornerstone of non-operative management in duodenal trauma are nil per os (NPO) with nasogastric tube (NGT) decompression, close monitoring with serial abdominal exams, serum amylase, lipase and follow-up CT scan in 12-24 h if clinical suspicion or deterioration [3].

In patients with hematoma and signs of obstruction, NOM is appropriate up to 14 days and should be taken to the OR to drain the hematoma if clinical deterioration, worsening findings on interval CT or to relieve the mechanical obstruction [3, 9, 10].

2.4.2 Operative management

During surgery, the decision to proceed with definitive repair versus damage-control and delayed repair is an important one, taking into account the high rate of complex or combined injuries, frequently resulting in hemorrhagic shock. During damage-control laparotomy, the aim is to achieve contamination control, often with primary suture repair, drainages and sometimes externally drain the bile duct.

Once adequate [11] resuscitation and hemodynamic stability is established in the intensive care unit, assessment of a definitive repair is considered at a second-look surgery [10].

Assessment of duodenal injuries is often made possible during surgery. Up to 55–85% of duodenal injuries can be managed by primary closure [1–3, 10]. Primary suture repair should be the initial approach in most situations, with more complex repairs reserved for extensive injuries. High-grade injuries are those which involve >75% of duodenal wall, D1 or D2 injuries, delayed repair and associated biliary or pancreatic injuries [2]. Injuries at D1 or proximal D2 can benefit from performing an antrectomy and Billroth II reconstruction [3].

Almost all grade I-II hematomas diagnosed pre-operatively resolve with adequate non-operative management. If hematomas are discovered during surgery and > 50% of lumen is compromised, it should be externally drained without entering the duodenal lumen. A gastrojejunostomy should be considered in case the hematoma compromises >75% of the lumen due to the risk of delayed obstruction [10]. Simple grade I and early grade II lacerations are managed by simple, tension-free repair with imbricating sutures in a transverse orientation and ensuring viable edges [3, 10]. Drains should not be routinely placed for Grade I-II injuries [9].

Up to 30% of duodenal injuries will require complex repair techniques [12]. Delayed or contaminated grade II injuries may be managed as grade III injuries. This often requires to perform a roux-en Y duodeno-jejunostomy in cases of extensive defects (grade III) [10] or grade II injuries where a tension-free repair is not possible or in some cases with moderate contamination [1].

Grade III injuries involving D1, D3 or D4 may likely undergo primary repair alone [11]. Extensive duodenal lacerations in D2-D3 segments may be repaired by an end-to-end duodenoduodenostomy [3]. Grade III-IV injuries not involving the ampulla or bile duct, benefit from the same approach as Grade III injuries [4, 9]. Small bowel anastomosis has an overall 9% complication rate. In trauma patients undergoing damage-control surgery, a delayed anastomosis shows comparable complication rates to those undergoing single-stage anastomosis [13].

Grade IV-V injuries are devastating, the patient often presents in hemorrhagic shock and usually requires a complex reconstruction technique [4]. These patients present with injuries involving the duodenopancreatic complex and often benefit from a damage-control surgery and a second-look surgery for a definitive repair or reconstruction. Surgical approaches range from surgical techniques used in grade III injuries such as duodeno-jejunostomy, or even performing a Whipple procedure if extensive duodenal devascularization or pancreatic head destruction is present [2, 10].

Pancreaticoduodenectomy (Whipple procedure), is indicated for injuries in the pancreatic head, duodenum, distal common bile duct, massive hemorrhage of difficult control and combined grade V pancreatic and duodenal injuries [1]. Reimplantation of the common bile duct into the duodenum carries a high risk of stricture formation [3]. In patients with destructive pancreatic injuries, anastomotic leaks are to be expected, thus external drainage of the anastomosis is vital for leakage control and enabling the formation of a controlled fistula [3].

2.4.2.1 Duodenal diversion

Procedures that divert enteric contents away from the duodenum may be considered in cases of high-grade injuries. All duodenal diversion techniques have similar complication and mortality rates. Their goal is to divert gastric contents and, in some situations, bilio/pancreatic contents from the duodenum to minimize the possibility of suture dehiscence, leakage and contamination.

2.4.2.2 Pyloric exclusion

Developed in 1977 by Vaughn et al., it consists of primary repair of the duodenum and diverting the gastric contents to the jejunum. After the duodenal repair, the pylorus is closed from the inside through a gastrotomy by means of suture or staples. The final step is to perform a gastrojejunostomy at the site of the gastrotomy [10]. The pylorus reopens spontaneously at 3 weeks, but the main long-term complication is an anastomotic ulcer in up to 33% of patients [10, 14]. Overall complication rates are higher in these patients (71%) [3].

2.4.2.3 Duodenostomy tube

This method of diversion consists in creating a lateral or end-tube duodenostomy near the injury site in cases where the degree of inflammation hinders any other approach.

2.4.2.4 Duodenal Diverticulization

This historic technique described by Berne et al. [15] was employed in cases of complex duodenal injuries and its principle is to divert all gastric and biliary secretions from the duodenum. It consists of primary repair of the duodenal injury, antrectomy, vagotomy, closure of duodenal stump over a decompressive end duodenostomy, placement of a T-tube in the common bile duct and periduodenal drains [10].

2.5 Nutrition

Early enteral feeding improves complications and mortality in critically ill trauma patients [16]. A greater benefit associated with early enteral nutrition is reported once the patient's hemodynamic stability has been established [10]. Feeding jejunostomy is an excellent way of accomplishing early enteral feeding after major trauma [10], especially in patients with severe pancreaticoduodenal injuries requiring resection and reconstruction [9]. Up to 75% of critically ill patients with severe duodenal injuries do not tolerate early enteral feeding even with concurrent decompression and feeding jejunostomy [16], this being the reason why 37–75% of patients may still require total parenteral nutrition [9].

2.6 Complications

Mortality ranges from 15 to 47% [3], many of them attributed to the associated injuries, especially major vascular injuries causing hemorrhagic shock [3]. In-hospital mortality and postoperative sepsis is similar in patients with primary-repair compared with gastrojejunostomy (6.6% vs. 4.5% and 10.4 vs. 6.7% respectively), but hospital length of stay is shorter in the primary repair group (11 days vs. 18 days) [17].

Overall complications reach 65% and include intra-abdominal abscess and sepsis, duodenal leakage (0–33%), bowel obstruction, and complications related to other injuries [3, 11]. Patients with severe intestinal injuries are at higher risk of intestinal leaks, perforation, volvuli and bowel necrosis [16]. Hypotension in both the preoperative and intraoperative period is the primary risk factor for complications [14].

Other risk factors include blunt abdominal trauma, high-speed projectiles, high-grade duodenal injuries, associated biliary tree injuries or severe pancreatic injuries and more than 24-hour delay in treatment [4, 18]. And some physiological measures associated with complications include lactate and pH level [19].

Intra-abdominal abscess presents with clinical deterioration between 7 to 10 days post-injury. Antibiotics and percutaneous drainage remain the standard of care [3].

Duodenal leak and fistula rates vary according to AAST injury grade and the affected duodenal segment. The more severe the injury, the higher risk of duodenal leak. AAST Grade I injuries have a risk of about 0% of leakage, AAST-II 1.6% and AAST III 66.7%. [19]. According to the affected segment, the risk of duodenal leak is 32% in D1, 12.5% in D2, 38.5% in D3 and 16% in D4 [19]. Factors that may enhance the risk of suture failure include distal intestinal obstruction and pancreatic injury with enzyme leaks.

The mainstay of treatment is adequate drainage, output control, maintaining euvolemia, replacing electrolytes losses and adequate nutrition [3]. Also, decompression of the bile and pancreatic secretions produced daily reduces the risk of duodenal leakage [11].

3. Conclusion

Duodenal injuries are often associated with other organ injuries, thus delaying diagnosis in some cases and increasing the risk of complication. When diagnosed in time, it can be treated with relatively low mortality rates.

There are several surgical techniques described to treat high-grade duodenal injuries, some of which are more complex than others, however, it is evident that primary closure has been superior in terms of results, inferring that it is less complex and with shorter surgical time. Outcomes are good, and the prognosis is tightly ligated to associated injuries, thus high index of suspicion and applying ATLS and surgery trauma principles are essential.

Based on the premise set forth by the Pan American Trauma Society, primary closure is postulated as the treatment of choice in duodenal trauma regardless of its grade; taking as a reference the adequate optimization of surgical times that allow the prompt resolution of the acute event, reducing the patient's exposure to metabolic response to trauma induced during the intervention; systematically resolving the patient's determinant of morbidity and mortality. This precept is mostly applicable in cases that present with hemodynamic instability. In addition, it is suggested that alternative procedures such as pyloric exclusion and/or additional decompression should be reserved for special cases [14].

Acknowledgements

All authors attest that they meet the current ICMJE criteria for Authorship.

Funding

This research did not receive any specific grant from funding agencies in the public, commercial, or not-for-profit sectors.

Conflict of interest

The authors declare no conflict of interest.

Author details

José Miguel Aceves-Ayala*, David Jacob Álvarez-Chávez,
Clara Elizabeth Valdez-Cruz, Cristhian Felipe Montoya-Salazar,
Carlos Alfredo Bautista-López, Cesar Alberto Ortiz-Orozco,
Wence Francisco Villalvazo-Zuñiga and Pablo Francisco Rojas-Solís
Civil Hospital of Guadalajara "Dr. Juan I. Menchaca", Guadalajara, México

*Address all correspondence to: josemiguelacevesayala@gmail.com

References

[1] Rickard MJFX, Brohi K, Bautz PC. Pancreatic and duodenal injuries: Keep it simple. ANZ Journal of Surgery. 2005;**75**:581-586. DOI: 10.1111/j.1445-2197.2005.03351.x

[2] García Santos E, Soto Sánchez A, Verde JM, Marini CP, Asensio JA, Petrone P. Lesiones duodenales secundarias a traumatismo: Revisión de la literatura. Cirugía Española. 2015;**93**:68-74. DOI: 10.1016/j.ciresp.2014.08.004

[3] Ratnasekera A, Ferrada P. Traumatic duodenal injury: Current management update. Current Surgery Reports. 2020;**8**:6. DOI: 10.1007/s40137-020-00251-9

[4] Magaña, Sánchez IJ, Manuel García Núñez L. Alternativas de manejo del trauma duodenal. Cirujano General. 2013;**34-37**

[5] Skandalakis JE, Colborn GL, Foster RS, Weidman TA, Skandalakis LJ, Skandalakis PN. Surgical Anatomy and Technique: A Pocket Manual. New York: Springer; 2002

[6] Melamud K, LeBedis CA, Soto JA. Imaging of pancreatic and duodenal trauma. Radiologic Clinics of North America. 2015;**53**:757-771. DOI: 10.1016/j.rcl.2015.02.009

[7] Velmahos GC. Blunt Pancreatoduodenal Injury a Multicenter Study of the Research Consortium of New England Centers for Trauma (ReCONECT). In: Archives of Surgery. American Medical Association (AMA). 2009;**144**(5):413. DOI: 10.1001/archsurg.2009.52

[8] Moore EE, Cogbill TH, Malangoni MA, Jurkovich GJ, Champion HR, Gennarelli TA, et al. Organ injury scaling, II: Pancreas, duodenum, small bowel, colon, and rectum. The Journal of Trauma. 1990;**30**:1427-1429

[9] Coccolini F, Kobayashi L, Kluger Y, Moore EE, Ansaloni L, Biffl W, et al. Duodeno-pancreatic and extrahepatic biliary tree trauma: WSES-AAST guidelines. World Journal of Emergency Surgery. 2019;**14**:1-23. DOI: 10.1186/S13017-019-0278-6

[10] Malhotra A, Biffl WL, Moore EE, Schreiber M, Albrecht RA, Cohen M, et al. Western trauma association critical decisions in trauma: Diagnosis and management of duodenal injuries. Journal of Trauma and Acute Care Surgery. 2015;**79**:1096-1101. DOI: 10.1097/TA.0000000000000870

[11] Schroeppel TJ, Saleem K, Sharpe JP, Magnotti LJ, Jordan AW, Fischer PE, et al. Penetrating duodenal trauma: A 19-year experience. Journal of Trauma and Acute Care Surgery. 2016;**80**:461-465. DOI: 10.1097/TA.0000000000000934

[12] Ferrada P, Wolfe L, Duchesne J, Fraga GP, Benjamin E, Alvarez A, et al. Management of duodenal trauma: A retrospective review from the Panamerican trauma society. Journal of Trauma and Acute Care Surgery. 2019;**86**:392-396. DOI: 10.1097/TA.0000000000002157

[13] Bruns BR. Bowel anastomosis in acute care surgery. Current Surgery Reports 2017;5, 29. doi:10.1007/s40137-017-0191-4

[14] Seamon MJ, Pieri PG, Fisher CA, Gaughan J, Santora TA, Pathak AS, et al. A ten-year retrospective review: Does pyloric exclusion improve clinical

outcome after penetrating duodenal and combined pancreaticoduodenal injuries? Journal of Trauma - Injury, Infection and Critical Care. 2007;**62**:829-833. DOI: 10.1097/TA.0b013e318033a790

[15] Berne CJ, Donovan AJ, White EJ, Yellin AE. Duodenal "diverticulization" for duodenal and pancreatic injury. American Journal of Surgery. 1974;**127**:503-507. DOI: 10.1016/0002-9610(74)90305-5

[16] Dickerson RN, Voss JR, Schroeppel TJ, Maish GO, Magnotti LJ, Minard G, et al. Feasibility of jejunal enteral nutrition for patients with severe duodenal injuries. Nutrition. 2016;**32**:309-314. DOI: 10.1016/J.NUT.2015.08.026

[17] Siboni S, Benjamin E, Haltmeier T, Inaba K, Demetriades D. Isolated blunt duodenal trauma: Simple repair, Low Mortality. American Surgery. 2015;**81**:961-964. DOI: 10.1177/000313481508101010

[18] Talbot WA, Shuck JM. Retroperitoneal duodenal injury due to blunt abdominal trauma. The American Journal of Surgery. 1975;**130**:659-666. DOI: 10.1016/0002-9610(75)90416-X

[19] Weale RD, Kong VY, Bekker W, Bruce JL, Oosthuizen G v., Laing GL, et al. Primary repair of duodenal injuries: A retrospective cohort study from a major trauma Centre in South Africa. Scandinavian Journal of Surgery 2019;**108**:280-284. doi:10.1177/1457496918822620

Chapter 4

Ultrasound Empowered Trauma Management

Mohammad Meshkini

Abstract

Using ultrasound to empower the way of traumatic patient early and by-side management as its ability to discover what bare eyes and hands could not find out solely. The most known EFAST protocol for traumatic patients management may be extended more wisely by introducing the ultrasound probe(s) through a head-to-toe secondary survey and giving a better idea of what is going on with the patient before transferring him/her out of the emergency department and could save the time and the patient's condition. This chapter would summarize what we know about ultrasound application on a traumatic patient by his/her side before sending him/her out for any further investigation, a new point of care for the standard of patient management by ultrasound.

Keywords: ultrasound, sonography, RUSH, POCUS, EFAST

1. Introduction

Observation has been one of the essentials of the clinical examination that can be found in almost every medical textbook. The use of various examination equipment due to the development of technology has improved clinical examinations and patient care. For example, we can mention the history of the invention of the stethoscope. Before the stethoscope was produced, physicians used to place their ears directly on the patient's body for auditory examinations, which was sometimes beyond the considerations of society; for this purpose, the first tool was made of a piece of paper, and later, better and advanced types were prepared, produced, and distributed.

It was mentioned the necessity of observation as one of the first steps of examining people; the possibility of using ultrasound to examine the internal organs of the body makes this purpose possible for a physician to observe and examine the inside of the patient's body by using an ultrasound probe even before auscultation, palpation, and percussion. By using ultrasound, the examiner can make a better clinical diagnosis of the patient. Also, due to the low invasiveness of this technology, it is possible to use it near the patient and reduce the complications caused by the clinical procedures, e.g., the success of the venipuncture with the use of ultrasound is more than the usual IV cannulation [1–4].

In this chapter, we will refer to the various applications of ultrasound from the perspective of its use in the management and treatment of trauma patients. And for detailed consideration, the tutorial videos are referenced from Youtube and Aparat streaming channels.

2. Orientation to the machine and probes

Proper recognition of a tool will make its use much more effective and efficient. For a more detailed understanding of the possible software and hardware features of the device, one should get familiar with the machine's instruction manual. However, in this chapter, we will discuss how to properly place the probes on the patient's body and the general tips for using medical ultrasound machines.

The ultrasound device's probes with an indicator will determine whether we should approach the patient. The placement of the piezoelectric crystals on the probe is in the same direction, and this will create only one row of sound that is interpreted by the operator in the plane of axial, coronal, or sagittal images (**Figures 1** and **2**).

At the beginning and for a general purpose, like other standard radiological images, the right side of the patient must be on the right side of the screen. For this purpose, the indicator is placed on the patient's right side and the resulting image is interpreted. On the other hand, if a coronal or sagittal view is needed, the indicator is placed toward the patient's head, which makes the image from the head toward the patient's feet.

Three common probes are:

- High-frequency Linear
- Low-frequency Convex
- Phased-Array (Echo), which is also a low-frequency probe

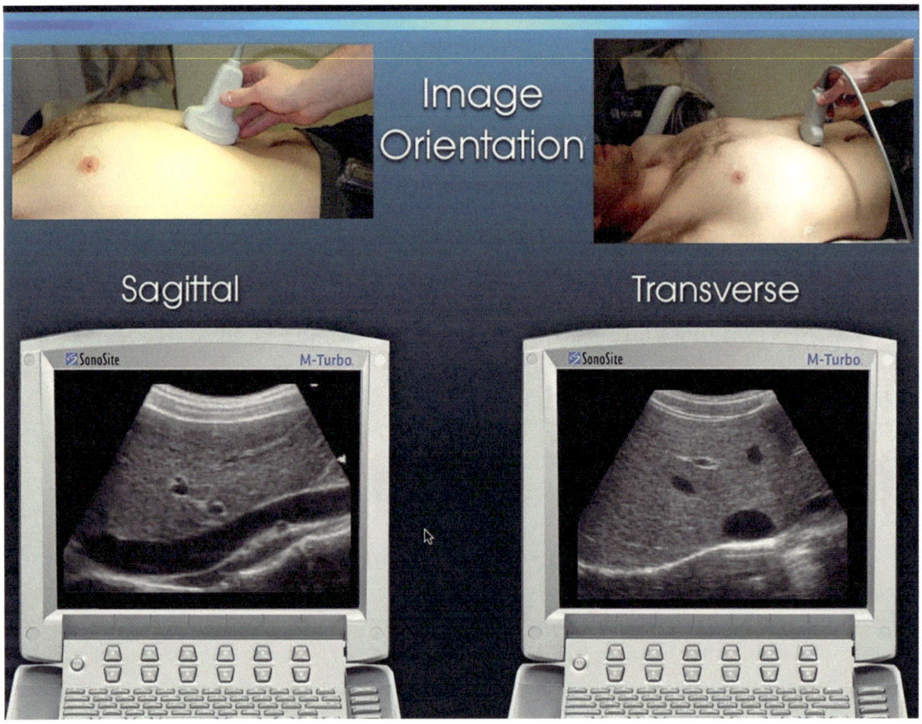

Figure 1.
How the image changes with different positioning of the probe (Courtesy of Dr. John Christian Fox).

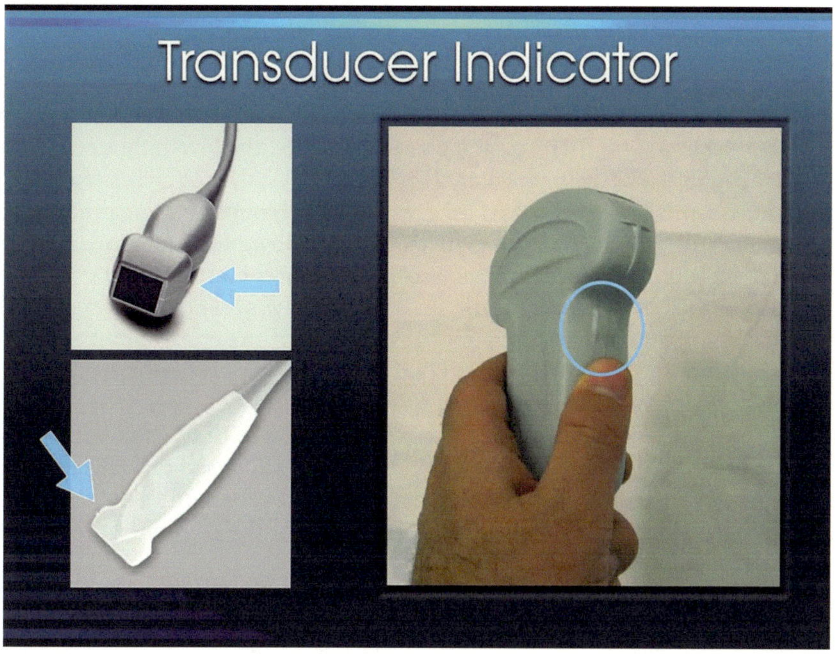

Figure 2.
Probes' indicators (Courtesy of Dr. John Christian Fox).

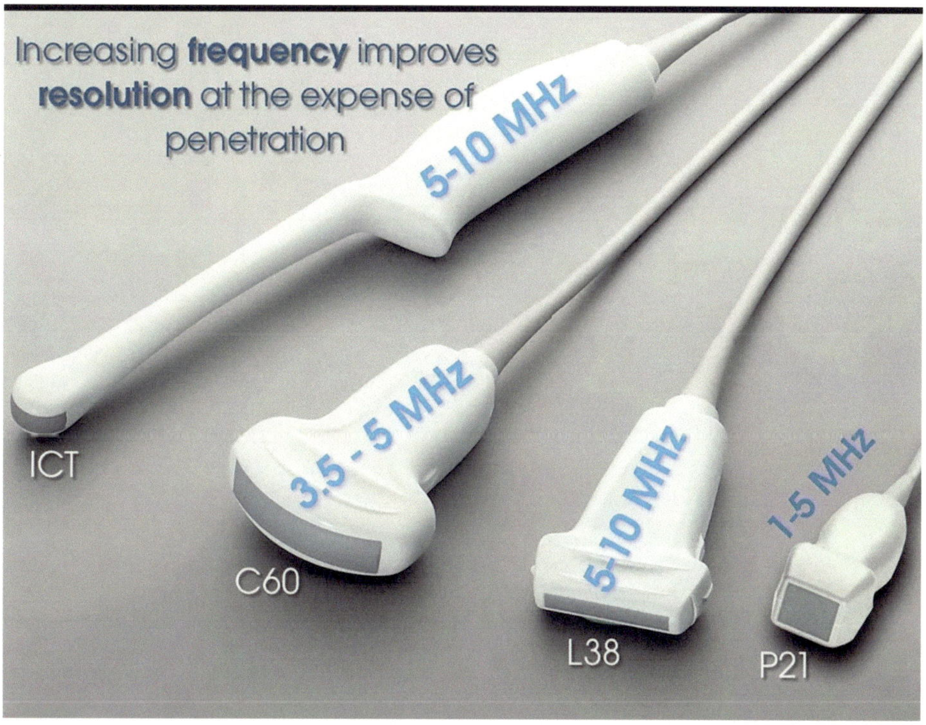

Figure 3.
Diverse types of probes (Courtesy of Dr. John Christian Fox).

A little physics of wave may be useful here; as the wave moves in the surrounding medium (environment), they have interactions with each other; the medium may reflect, absorb, or pass (with some changes) the wave, and what we see on the ultrasound machine's screen are those reflected from the medium. The body as a medium may absorb most of the high-frequency waves; however, the low-frequency waves may travel through the body more easily (**Figure 3**).

The air and bone are the two most reflective media (sound waves cannot penetrate them and may reflect through making an acoustic shadow phenomenon); however, other media (such as musculature, fat, fibro-skeletal, and internal solid organs) may pass the wave with some interactions on its amplitude (power) or velocity (speed); however, water and liquid may pass almost every part of the wave but when the wave reaches to the other medium due to media difference, it may get reflected and make acoustic echo phenomenon (**Figures 4–6**).

Though the high-frequency probes are used for surface study, their wave cannot penetrate deep into the body. But low-frequency probes are used for deeper studies. However, some use low-frequency convex probes for surface studies by reducing their penetrating depth, it may speed up their examination of the patient but could not display the detailed view like a high-frequency probe can.

By the way, the higher frequency of a wave makes it for better images, (e.g., 60 Hz vs. 90 Hz vs. 120 Hz commercial displays may be a good example of image sharpness and brings this topic to mind) (Video 1, https://www.youtube.com/watch?v=VBHCmw8iHCc&list=PL539B142177BA83F7, https://www.aparat.com/v/9ifZw).

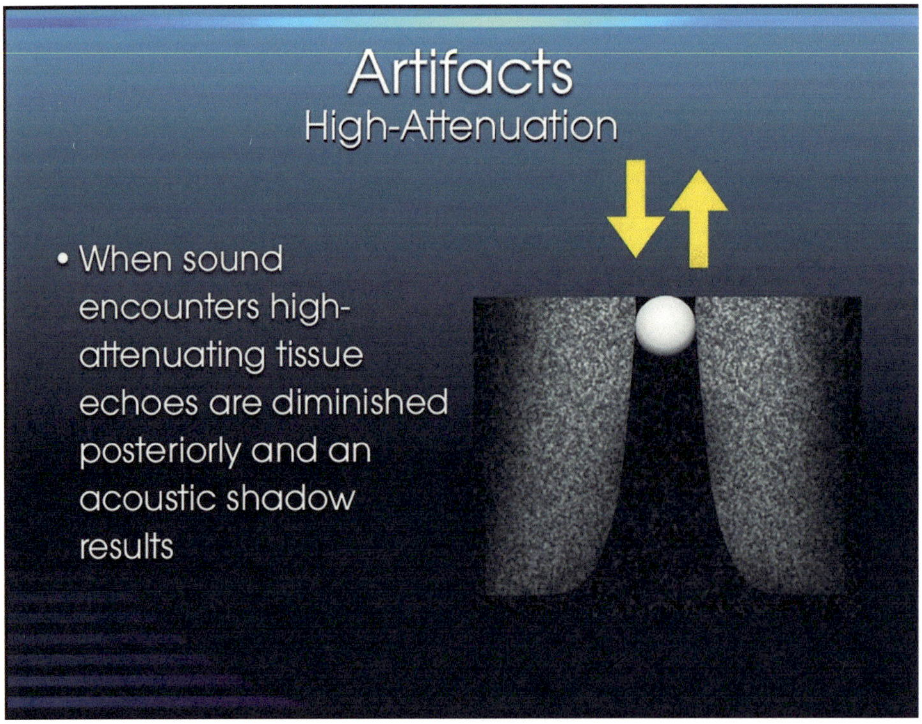

Figure 4.
Posterior shadow (Courtesy of Dr. John Christian Fox).

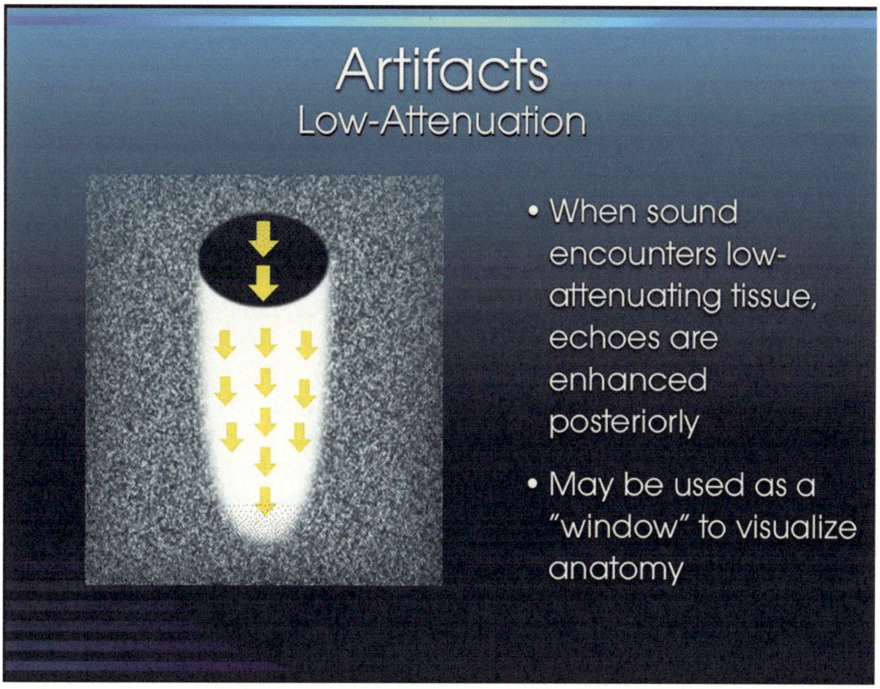

Figure 5.
Posterior echo (Courtesy of Dr. John Christian Fox).

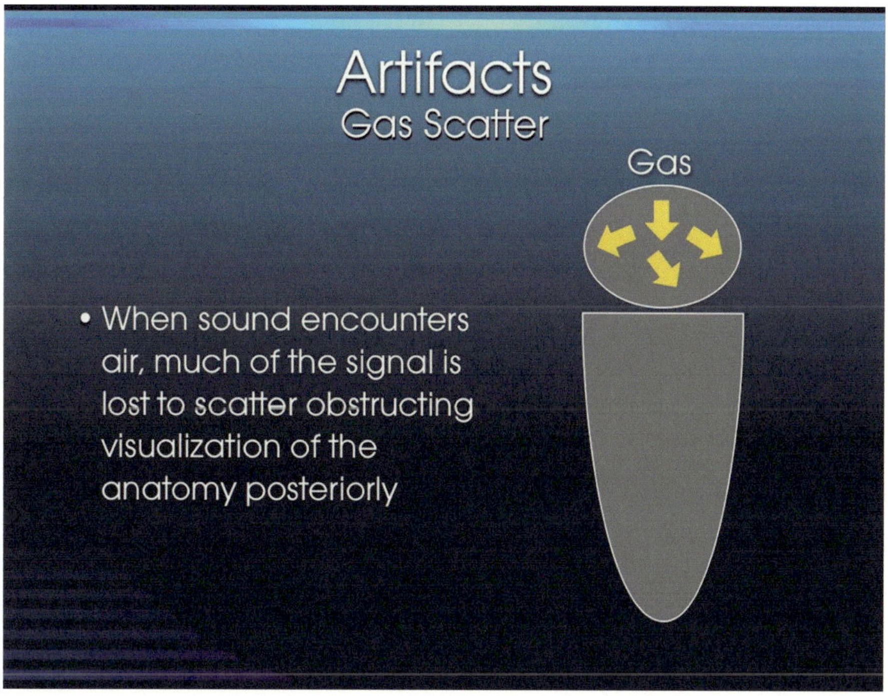

Figure 6.
Gas scattering (Courtesy of Dr. John Christian Fox).

3. Empowering airway assessment

Guidelines of the ATLS emphasize on airway as a priority in the ABCDE approach; for airway assessment other than using LEMON criteria, the ultrasound could be used for further evaluation and even intubation confirmation; however, as ultrasound is non-penetrating through the air, it may be out of mind. Here's how we could use ultrasound for assessing airway:

For assessing the larynx and its cartilages, put the linear probe with the indicator pointing to the patient's head on the anterior cervical mid-line. A white line should be observed, which may show the triangular shape on the beginning and right side of the screen, it is the thyroid cartilage, above this structure (right side of the screen), the hyoid bone (and vocal cords) could be studied, and beneath the thyroid cartilage is the place for cricoid and three or four tracheal rings (above manubrium), the thyroid gland, which is a normo-echoic structure, is placed superficial to these beneath structures.

By turning the probe's indicator to the right side, it provides axial plane images from the body, the vocal cords may be seen in this way more accurately; however, for evaluating and confirmation of the endo-tracheal tube (ETT) with ultrasound, the most specific approach is to not find it through the esophagus, which mostly lay right-posterior to the trachea. Also, the ETT has air inside the tube and reflects the ultrasound wave in a scattering pattern (Video 2, https://www.aparat.com/v/0cZr5?t=638).

This method may also be useful in forecasting the size of the trachea, ETT, and LMA size(s) too [5].

4. Empowering breathing assessment

As lung ultrasound was introduced with BLUE protocol about 10–15 years ago, it could even change the FAST exam into E-FAST [6]. However, searching for

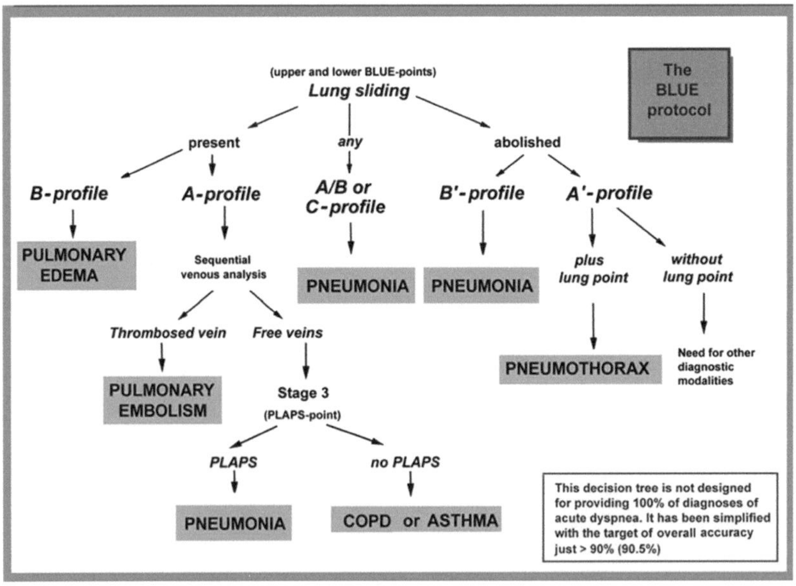

Figure 7.
BLUE-protocol algorithm.

pneumothoraces or hemothoraces is not the only application of the lung ultrasound, searching for rocket b-lines (b-lines that extend more deep in the field), vascular profile, etc., may help the physician for diagnosing the probable reasons for the acute respiratory failure (**Figure 7** and Video 3, https://www.youtube.com/watch?v=RFrPO-8jQP4&list=PL2AGl6-lzXJQt3LGH0Fqc5rjIn_hwmfhZ, https://www.aparat.com/v/aqSYt?t=664). Because it's out of consideration for trauma management, we leave it for your own for further investigation. The latest chest journal paper in 2015 is highly recommended [7]. Also the E-FAST and RUSH protocols are covered in the circulation section.

5. Empowering circulation assessment

The Focused Abdominal Sonography for Trauma (FAST) was first introduced to get a surrogate for Deep Peritoneal Lavage (DPL), it covered only three windows: right-side hepato-renal (Morrison Punch), left-side splenorenal, and supra-pubic peri-vesical views. Then it has been changed into Focused Assessment Sonography for Trauma (FAST) due to the advancement of the 4th window, Sub-Xiphoid pericardial assessment, and nowadays the Extended-Focused Assessment Sonography for Trauma(E-FAST) protocol took place for this purpose by assessing for the pneumothorax and hemothorax [6, 8].

To cover this examination by patient side, mostly we start with a low-frequency probe (To reduce the effects of ribs concealing shadows, most experts use a phased-array probe rather than a convex probe.) from the right hepatorenal side putting the probe in the

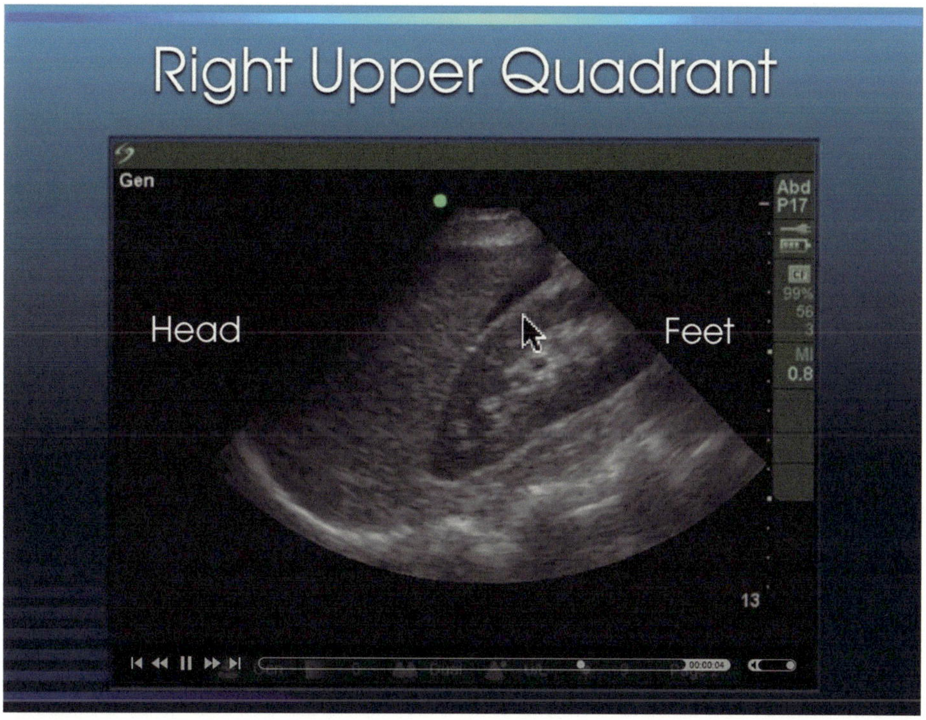

Figure 8.
A positive FAST exam on right hepatorenal (Courtesy of Dr. John Christian Fox).

sagittal plane of the right mid-axillary and beneath 7-8th inter-costal space, indicator of which lays toward the head of the patient; some fanning also could be helpful to find out the right kidney, and the Morrison punch is the potential space between right kidney and the liver, if any kind of fluid (a dark hypoechoic media with bright posterior acoustic echo) may be observed in this place, it would be positive FAST and needs surgical considerations. It's recommended to not lose as much information as needed and to set the depth of examination up to the posterior spinal column (**Figure 8**).

Like the right side, the examination of the splenorenal in the left needs the same approach; however, the left spleen mostly is posterior and superior, which needs probe positioning in the left mid to posterior axillary line and sometimes full inspiration of the patient to the full view of the space (**Figure 9**).

For studying the suprapubic perivesical site, put the probe with the indicator toward the right side of the body just above the pubic symphysis and slightly tilt and fan the probe toward the pelvic, the bladder will come out as a pouch full of fluid, for determining whether there is any free fluid around the bladder, the most specific site is its posterior (Douglas pouch in female, and also posterior to the womb is potential to get fluid in there); for this goal, just tilt the probe somehow to see the posterior part of the bladder better and then change it into coronal position as the indicator toward the head, this maneuver will change the operator's point of view from axial into coronal and the posterior side of the bladder may come into the field better, i.e., what is shown on the right side of the screen (probe is indicating toward the head) is lay on the posterior side of the bladder (**Figure 10**).

Meanwhile, the sub-xiphoid pericardial view is the 4th side of the classic FAST, in case it could not achievable, some recommend for left sternal border window for

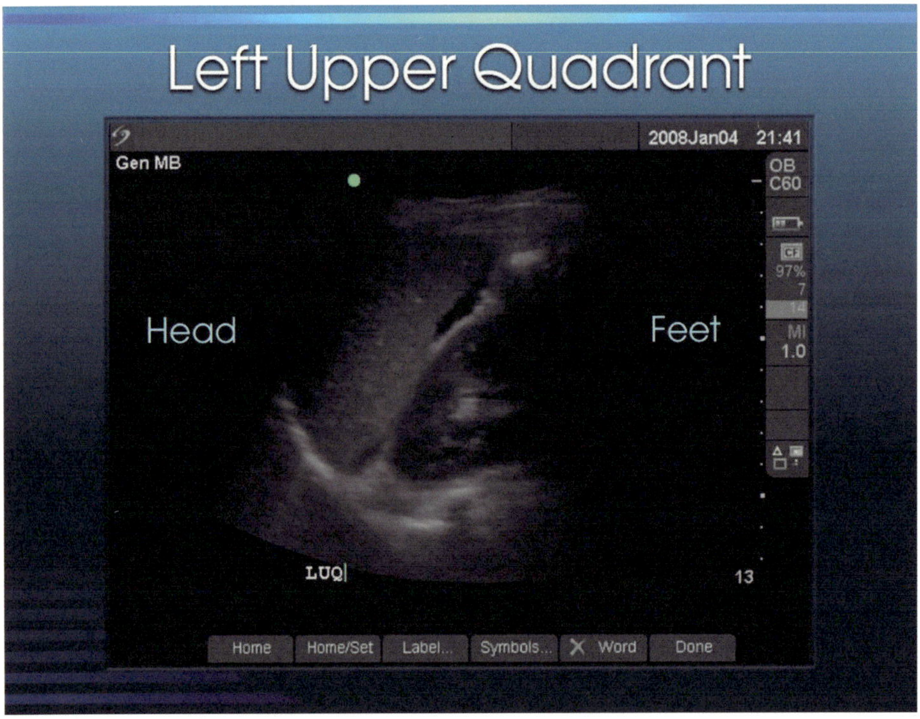

Figure 9.
A positive FAST exam on left splenorenal (Courtesy of Dr. John Christian Fox).

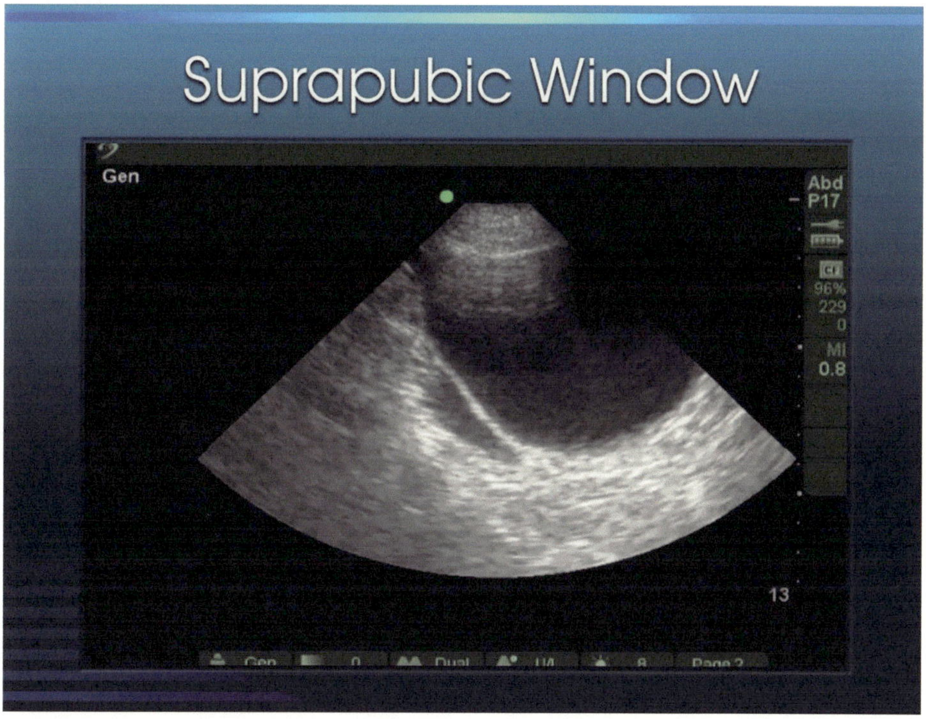

Figure 10.
A positive FAST exam on suprapubic perivesial (Courtesy of Dr. John Christian Fox).

this goal. However, before starting from the sub-xiphoid, increase the depth of the machine for more than 20 cm in an adult patient, put the probe with the indicator toward the right side, and try to open this window using the liver medium on the right side, because of the scattering phenomenon of the gastric gas that may obscure the field, if the image came out to study the heart as a four-chamber view with right ventricle, which lays on top of the liver (the chamber is near to the probe), the left ventricle is behind it on the screen, the right atrium is the chamber lays on the right side of the screen, and the left atrium is what leftover far from the probe (**Figure 11**). However, in case this image was not available, more pressure may be needed to better visualize the field, but some references prohibit it in children due to the probability of sudden cardiac arrest, at this time the parasternal view may be much more helpful.

After completing this four-site ultrasound examination, for extending the assessment for the trauma, it's time for assessing chest fields for possible pneumothorax or hemothorax. We would expect the gas to be higher and the liquid to be lower, so if pneumothorax is made, it could be on the anterior part of the chest. Using motion mode (M-Mode) should determine the pleural motion better than a normal lung sliding (or sea-shore sign) (**Figure 12**); however, in pneumothorax, this sliding is not shown because all of the points from the skin to the pleura are standstill (they do not move like normal lung movement), they demonstrate a stratosphere (or barcode) sign, by the way sometimes in pneumothoraces that does not fulfill the field, a lung point be may observed (**Figure 13**). For this purpose, use a high-frequency linear probe or decrease the depth of the curve probe, which was used during other parts of the FAST exam to 3–4 cm. Put the probe with the indicator toward the patient's head and start studying the lung for possible pneumothoraces on the anterior part of each

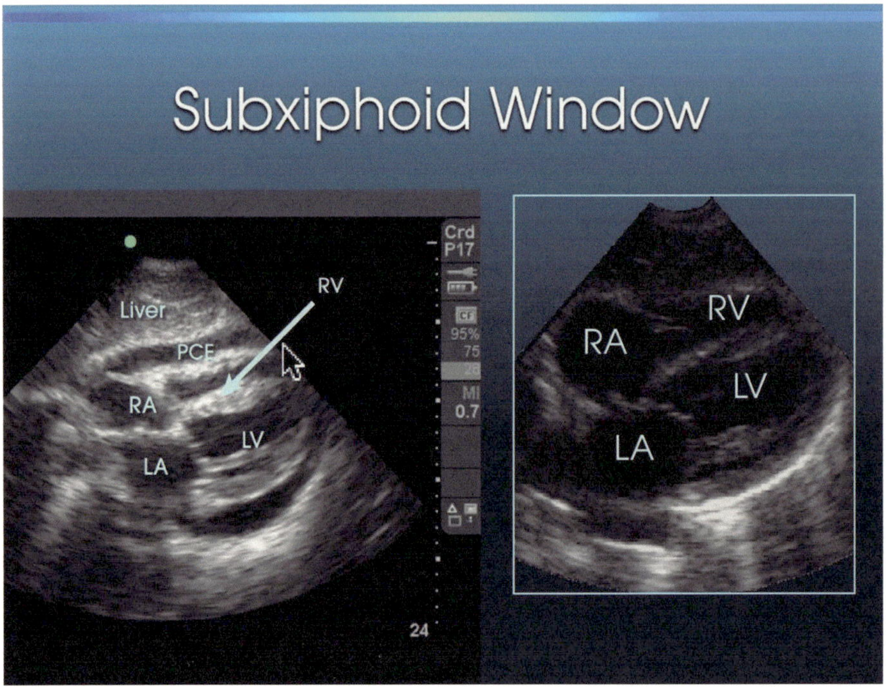

Figure 11.
A positive FAST exam as pericardial effusion (Courtesy of Dr. John Christian Fox).

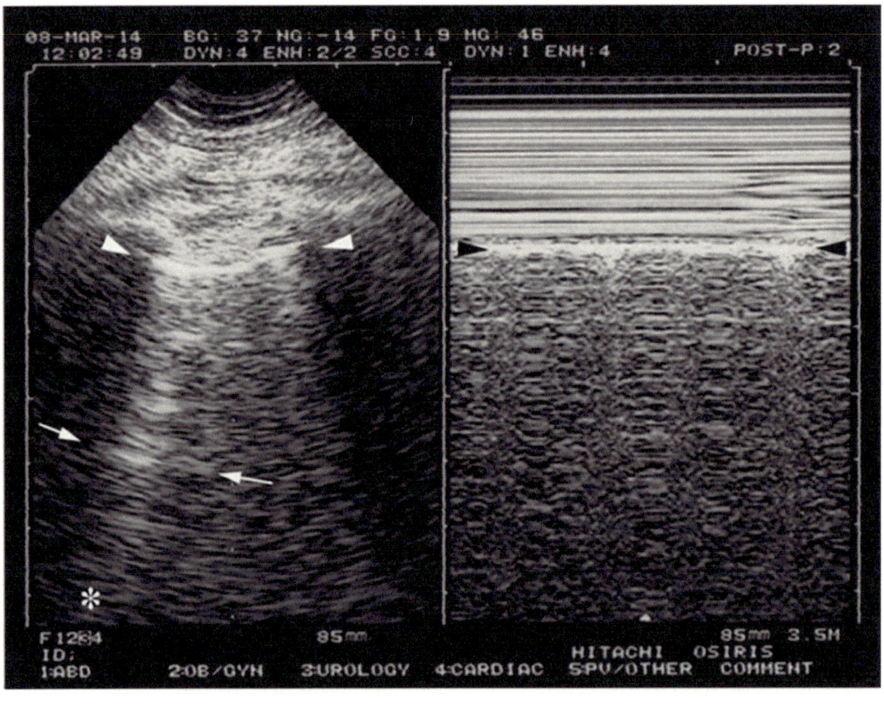

Figure 12.
Normal Lung-Sliding (Sea-Shore sign) (Courtesy of Daniel A. Lichtenstein).

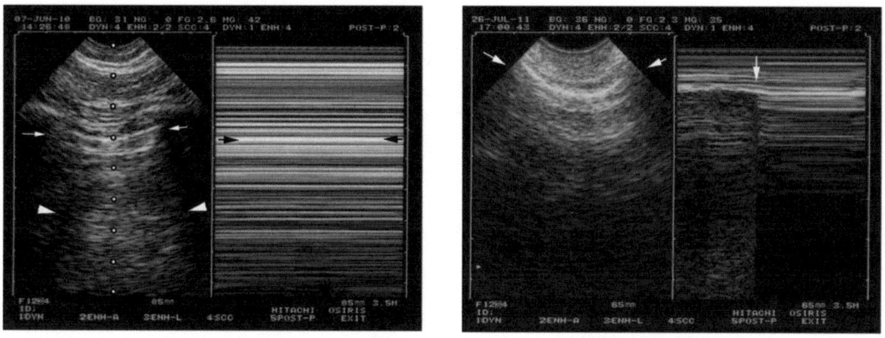

Figure 13.
Stratosphere & lung-point signs of pneumothorax (Courtesy of Daniel A. Lichtenstein).

side from the upper clavicular region up to down rib cages. For assessing the fluid (e.g., hemothorax or pleural effusion), the best place is superior to the diaphragm, where it's expected that the chest fluid may be stuck, it could also be examined while hepatorenal and splenorenal examination and considering diminished mirror effect of the diaphragm toward the head site. Video 4 (https://www.youtube.com/watch?v=klqeADRgvkM&list=PL2AGl6-lzXJTRn113DAv1Iybh_AFHBwFX, https://www.aparat.com/v/RBo4v) has a full list play of the E-FAST exam.

Even IV cannulation is much safer and easier with the power of ultrasound; however, in almost every procedure using ultrasound, two operators are recommended, the sono-expert to hold the probe and bring the good field of action, and the other operator to do the procedure. For this goal, first the vein should find in the axial plane and place the target in mid-line with the probe; measure the depth of the target from the skin (that probe lies on it), with the law of trigonometry in mind, presume an isosceles right triangle by manipulating the needle in the equal length of the target depth in a 45-degree angle. Change the probe position from axial, parallel to the needle that indicates toward needle (this maneuver shows all of the vein in a longitudinal view) and advance the needle then, popping into the vessel could also be seen on the screen, and cannulation is achieved [2]. This technique is the principal for almost every vascular cannulation or regional nerve block, Videos 5 (https://www.youtube.com/watch?v=uHfeyAYiWOc&list=PL9883F0497505F4B1, https://www.aparat.com/v/U1TA0?t=199), 6 (https://www.youtube.com/watch?v=EUMqxKJ2mPA&list=PL2AGl6-lzXJRBLHhfE-VsywsfUxqnHBHXG, https://www.aparat.com/v/0cZr5?t=807) and 14 (https://www.youtube.com/watch?v=ndnZxAcNjdg&list=PL09BFE9E4CB8A7050, https://www.youtube.com/watch?v=xvAY_bu_S7A&list=PL2AGl6-lzXJSYEVni4b7V8yAC8pmtccaX) are playlists of these procedures [3, 4, 9].

There's another ultrasound protocol for critical-care and hypotensive patients that is known as the RUSH exam, the Rapid Ultrasound for Shock and Hemorrhage [1, 10, 11]. It was first described in 2006 and got into medical literature 3–4 years by. Also, trauma patients may be in shock, and other than "Blood on the floor, and four/five more (Chest, Abdomen, Pelvic, Femur(long bones) and SCALP are potential sites for life-threatening bleeding)," a RUSH exam may empower the physicians' consideration on the possible reason of the shock (other than blood loss). The RUSH protocol divides the homeostatic system into "Pump," "Tank," and "Pipes." Which is an example of "Heart," "Potential spaces," and "Vessels," respectively.

Focused primary echocardiography could study the heart for its musculature and valve movements, their insufficiency could be obtained, and more results

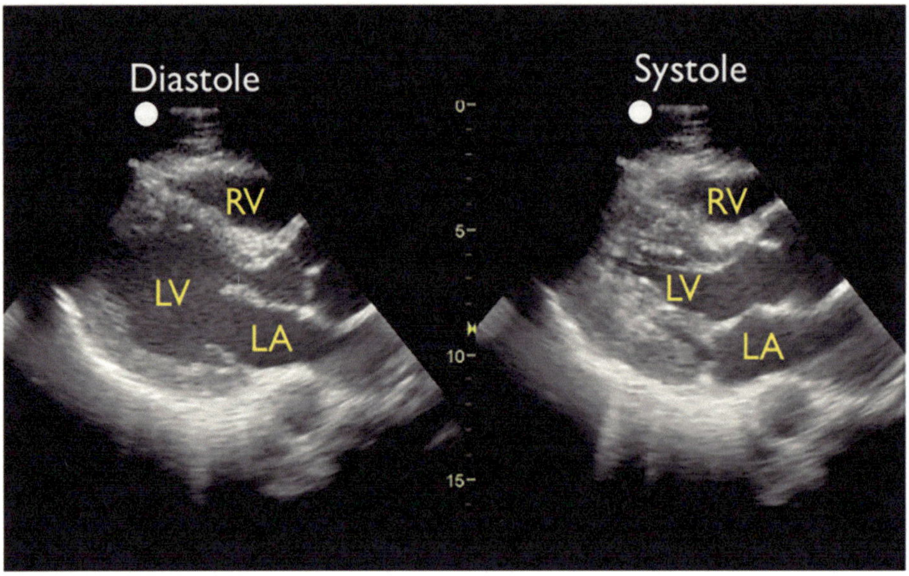

Figure 14.
Long-axis parasternal view.

could be achieved than just pericardial effusion purpose of the E-FAST exam. For this goal, start with the parasternal, then apical four-chamber, and finally the sub-xiphoid windows. On the long-axis parasternal the indicator of the probe toward the right shoulder, while on the short-axis parasternal, it aims at the left shoulder. The long-axis and short-axis views are demonstrated in **Figures 14** and **15** in systole and diastole, also ventricular contractility and LVEF could be obtained through this window using M-Mode, which is demonstrated in **Figure 16**. for achieving the apical view, put the probe on the Point of Maximum Impulse (PMI) on the left 5–6th mid-clavicular inter-costal space, both the probe and screen indicator should be in the same position (if it wasn't changed after the short-axis view, it's expected to be on the left side), what appear in the four-chamber view are two ventricles adjacent to the probe and two atria far from the probe, the right heart is on the right side and the left is on the left-side (pay attention to the probe and screen indicators' sameness), using Color-Doppler mode could bring the valves functionality and chambers' flow very well. And finally, the sub-xiphoid view, which is the standard recommended view in the FAST exam and was discussed there (Video 7, https://www.youtube.com/watch?v=1UJ6RodOSTw&list=PL2AGl6-lzXJRp3Dh0t1YZ2qsyic0msYDd, https://www.aparat.com/v/bmzqQ).

The "tank" or potential spaces are mostly covered by E-FAST examinations, the potential spaces for free fluid and great vessels like the Aorta and the IVC. The aorta and IVC both could be part of a cardiac exam too, thus they are great vessels of the body, in a shock patient, the aorta could be torn or aneurysmal, where both could be evaluated in descending abdominal aorta by using low-frequency convex or phased-array probe, both in axial and sagittal planes. Just it should be kept in mind that it may need extra force to pull over intestinal and gastric gas to find out vascular structures, also IVC lay just on the right side of the aorta and could be examined with the aorta or from the right hepatic window in sagittal plain (**Figure 17** and Video 8, https://www.youtube.com/

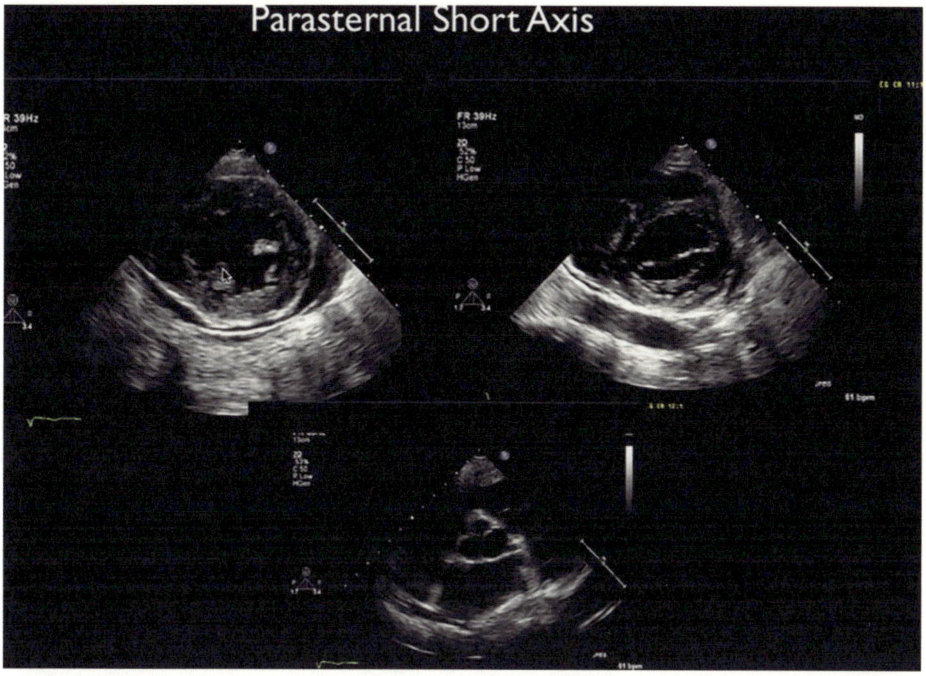

Figure 15.
Short-axis parasternal view for mitral valve (Courtesy of Dr. John Christian Fox).

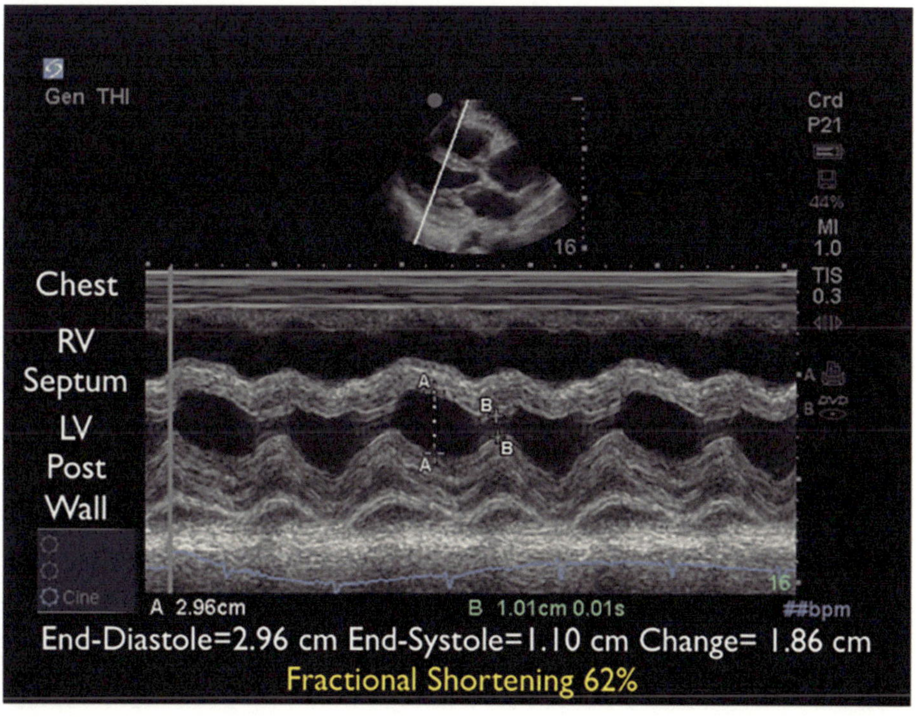

Figure 16.
Using M-mode for assessing contractility.

IVC Size	Respiratory Change	RA Pressure (cm)
<1.5	Total Collapse	0-5
1.5-2.5	>50% Collapse	5-10
1.5-2.5	<50% Collapse	11-15
>2.5	<50% Collapse	16-20
>2.5	None	>20

Figure 17.
IVC size and changes correlation with CVP.

watch?v=khD3dnxEt2o&list=PL2AGl6-lzXJRtdqShRXDozbmtx6Pw4fZC, https://www.aparat.com/v/bmzqQ?t=1247).

And finally, the "pipes" are mostly referred to deep veins for DVTs. The three-point access that consists of femoral, popliteal, and greater saphenous veins on each side is the acceptable examination for Deep Vein studies (Video 8, https://www.youtube.com/watch?v=khD3dnxEt2o&list=PL2AGl6-lzXJRtdqShRXDozbmtx6Pw4fZC, https://www.aparat.com/v/bmzqQ?t=1247).

All of these exams could be summarized as "HI MAP ED" mnemonic [11]:

	Step no. 1	Step no. 2	Step no. 3
Pump	Pericardial effusion: (a) Effusion present? (b) Signs of tamponade? Diastolic collapse of R Vent +/− R Atrium?	Left ventricular contractility: (a) Hyperdynamic? (b) Normal? (c) Decreased?	Right ventricular strain: (a) Increased size of RV? (b) Septal displacement from right to left?
Tank	Tank volume: (1) Inferior vena cava: (a) Large size/small Insp collapse? —CVP high— (b) Small size/large Insp collapse? —CVP Low— (2) Internal jugular veins: (a) Small or large?	Tank leakiness: (1) E-FAST exam: (a) Free fluid Abd/Pelvis? (b) Free fluid thoracic cavity? (2) Pulm edema: Lung rockets?	Tank compromise: Tension pneumothorax? (a) Absent lung sliding? (b) Absent comet tails?
Pipes	Abdominal aorta aneurysm: Abd aorta > 3 cm?	Thoracic aorta aneurysm/dissection: (a) Aortic root > 3.8 cm? (b) Intimal flap? (c) Thor aorta > 5 cm?	(1) Femoral vein DVT? Noncompressible vessel? (2) Popliteal vein DVT? Noncompressible vessel?

Figure 18.
Using the RUSH protocol to diagnose the type of shock.

RUSH exam	Hypovolemic shock	Cardiogenic shock	Obstructive shock	Distributive shock
Pump	Hypercontractile heart Small heart size	Hypocontractile heart Dilated heart size	Pericardial effusion, RV strain Hypercontractile heart	Hypercontractile heart (early sepsis) Hypocontractile heart (late sepsis)
Tank	Flat IVC Flat IJV Peritoneal fluid Pleural fluid	Distended IVC Distended IJV Lung rockets Pleural effusions, ascites	Distended IVC Distended IJV Absent lung sliding (PTX)	Normal/small IVC Normal/small IJV Pleural fluid (empyema) Peritoneal fluid (peritonitis)
Pipes	AAA Aortic dissection	Normal	DVT	Normal

Figure 19.
RUSH protocol summary.

- Heart
- IVC
- Morrison pouch and complete FAST exam
- Aorta
- Pleural space and pneumothorax
- Ectopic pregnancy (Video 13, https://www.youtube.com/watch?v=GBpiF7ML1CA&list=PL2AGl6-lzXJT4sk_DMVQtBNapC36AgTZp, https://www.aparat.com/v/ukBwf)
- DVTand the final diagnosis of shock reason could get whether the "pump," "tank," or "pipes" are responsible; **Figures 18** and **19** summarize the RUSH protocol (Video 9, https://www.youtube.com/watch?v=9UyVHqvGgHE&list=PL2AGl6-lzXJS9fkywFRsQIwzp31-Lc1nX, https://www.aparat.com/v/zEvcw).

6. Empowering diagnosis and neurological assessment

The high-frequency linear probe could be used for skin and soft tissue examination, e.g., cellulitis and soft tissue infection's cobblestone pattern (Video 12, https://www.aparat.com/v/U1TA0?t=71). Using this probe also could be the on-site tool for assessing tendons and muscles movements, bone fractures (also to assess whether fracture bone has been reduced after manipulation), and other orthopedic examinations (Video 11, https://www.youtube.com/watch?v=7G56DN38mz8&list=PLEF41F6DAEE3FD1A8, https://www.aparat.com/v/0cZr5?t=5). As described in IV canulation, the regional nerve block could be done using ultrasound power though with fewer complications (Video 14, https://www.youtube.com/watch?v=ndnZxAcNjdg&list=PL09BFE9E4CB8A7050, https://www.youtube.com/watch?v=xvAY_bu_S7A&list=PL2AGl6-lzXJSYEVni4b7V8yAC8pmtccaX).

However, ocular ultrasound may be the indescribable use of the linear probe in the emergency department, other than studying the orbit structure for lens and retinal placement or detachments, Iris muscles movement and pupil reflex, and anterior and posterior chambers of the eyeball, the rise of Intra Cranial Pressure (ICP) could affect optic nerve (Cranial Nerve II) and widen its diameter, this could be assessed after freezing the image on the screen and measuring the optic nerve's external diameter in 3 mm length to the orbit entrance, whether this sheath is more than 5 mm

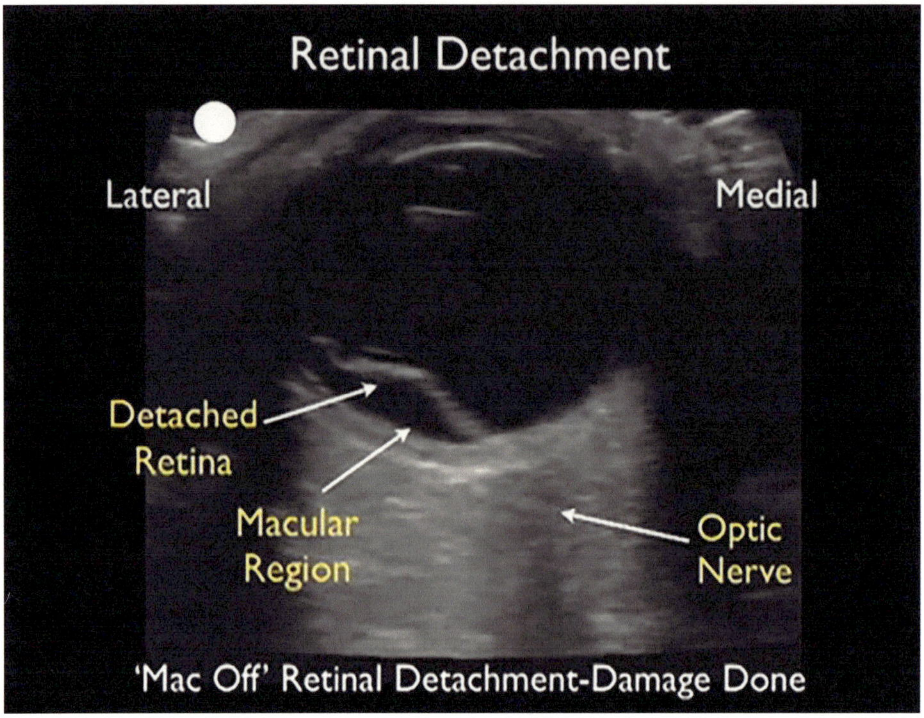

Figure 20.
Retinal detachment in occular B-mode ultrasound.

in diameter length it shows a rise in ICP, **Figure 20** shows retinal detachment, while other ocular ultrasound anatomical structures (Video 10, https://www.youtube.com/watch?v=uPqTz4OuNd0&list=PL2AGl6-lzXJTPj1GxVxCVyeg_srRs7oVg, https://www.aparat.com/v/0cZr5?t=235).

7. Conclusions

Using ultrasound alongside clinical examinations or during critical-care procedures empowers the ability of healthcare providers and physicians for better clinical decision makings and less invasive procedures. Like other clinical procedures, those who try and study more on the ultrasound could achieve better results, we recommend the use of ultrasound in any possible clinical situation for all providers, and the links that are mentioned in the appendices are highly recommended for reference.

Acknowledgements

I would like to mention the support and consideration of my kind family, especially my lovely wife who has always been there; besides, I need to acknowledge all my colleagues in the emergency department of Imam Khomeini hospital, Sarab, Iran; specifically the ward supervisor Mr. Masoud Abeshzadeh, ward-nurses Mrs. Feyzi, Mr. Reza Sayyareh, Mr. Mohammad Shokri, and my supportive alumni Dr. Roghayyeh Yaghoubi and Dr. Saba Nemati, for all of their kind and support during working shifts and recording tutorial videos. Also, I have to greet whoever tries to make the knowledge and experience sharing free and achievable for all around the world, especially "InTech Open" and "Free Software Foundation."

Conflict of interest

There is no conflict of interest to report.

Acronyms and abbreviations

ACS	American College of Surgeons
ACLS	Advanced Cardiac Life Support
AHA	American Heart Association
ATLS	Advanced Trauma Life Support
BLUE	Bedside Lung Ultrasound in Emergency department
COT	Committee On Trauma
DVT	Deep Vein Thrombosis
EFAST	Extended Focused Assessment Sonography for Trauma
ETT	Endo Tracheal Tube
ICP	Intra Cranial Pressure
IVC	Inferior Vena Cava
LEMON	Look externally, Evaluate 3-3-2, Mallampati score, Obstruction, Neck mobility
LMA	Laryngeal Mask Airway
PMI	Point of Maximum Impluse
POCUS	Point Of Care UltraSound
RUSH	Rapid Ultrasound in Shock and Hemorrhage

Appendices and nomenclature

1. https://www.aparat.com/v/9ifZw?playlist=1629800 (My Aparat.com channel's playlist for Ultrasound Tutor—In Persian Language).

2. https://www.youtube.com/c/sonosite (Fujifilm—Sonosite Youtube! Channel).

3. https://www.youtube.com/user/jfoxmd (Dr. John Christian Fox's Youtube! Channel).

Author details

Mohammad Meshkini[1,2]*

1 Road Traffic Injury Research Center (Tabriz International Safe Community Support Center), Tabriz University of Medical Sciences, Tabriz, Iran

2 Emergency Medicine Department, Sarab Faculty of Medical Sciences, Sarab, Iran

*Address all correspondence to: meshkini522@gmail.com

References

[1] Díaz-Gómez JL, Mayo PH, Koenig SJ. Point-of-care ultrasonography The New England Journal of Medicine 2021;**385**(17):1593-1602.

[2] Joing S, Strote S, Caroon L, Wall C, Hess J, Roline C, et al. Ultrasound-guided peripheral IV placement. The New England Journal of Medicine. 2012;**366**(25):e38

[3] Schulman PM, Gerstein NS, Merkel MJ, Braner DA, Tegtmeyer K. Ultrasound-guided cannulation of the subclavian vein. The New England Journal of Medicine. 2018;**379**(1):e1

[4] Ortega R, Song M, Hansen CJ, Barash P. Ultrasound-guided internal jugular vein cannulation. The New England Journal of Medicine. 2010;**362**(16):e57

[5] Adi O, Kok MS, Abdull Wahab SF. Focused airway ultrasound: An armamentarium in future airway management. Journal of Emergency and Critical Care Medicine. 2019;**3**:31-31

[6] Canelli R, Leo M, Mizelle J, Shrestha GS, Patel N, Ortega R. Use of eFAST in patients with injury to the thorax or abdomen. The New England Journal of Medicine. 2022;**386**(10):e23

[7] Lichtenstein DA. BLUE-protocol and FALLS-protocol. Chest. 2015;**147**(6):1659-1670

[8] Chardouli M, Yasinzadeh M, Meshkini M, Jalilvand H, Basir Ghafouri H, Sadeghi-Bazargani H, et al. A review on using ultrasound for evaluation of pediatric blunt abdominal trauma. Frontiers in Emergency Medicine. 2021. Available from: https://publish.kne-publishing.com/index.php/FEM/article/view/7680

[9] Peris A, Tutino L, Cianchi G, Gensini G. Ultrasound guidance for pleural-catheter placement. The New England Journal of Medicine. 2018;**378**(14):e19

[10] Seif D, Perera P, Mailhot T, Riley D, Mandavia D. Bedside ultrasound in resuscitation and the rapid ultrasound in shock protocol. Critical Care Research and Practice. 2012;**2012**:1-14

[11] EmCrit Project. Rapid ultrasound for shock and hypotension. Available from: https://emcrit.org/rush-exam/original-rush-article/

Chapter 5

OCD of the Knee in Adolescents

Andrey Semenov, Dmitriy Vybornov, Nikolaj Tarasov, Vladimir Krestyashin, Ivan Isaev and Vladimir Koroteev

Abstract

Osteochondritis dissecans (OCD) of the knee is a pathological condition of subchondral bone resembling focal osteolysis with subsequent bone resorption, which may lead to osteochondral fragment separation. Several etiological concepts reported for OCD development. The multifactorial theory is commonly adopted for days. Different investigators report OCD lesion healing while using conservative treatment or even "waitful watching" with a healing rate of up to 67%. In spite of these results, there are not any commonly adopted guidelines for conservative treatment. The last stage of OCD is a separation of osteochondral fragment leaving a full-thickness osteochondral defect, which is usually filled with low-quality fibrocartilaginous tissue. This tissue provides a lesser extent of resistance to peak loading forces, which poses at risk subchondral bone for further destruction and early osteoarthritis development. Appropriate treatment method should be chosen for each OCD stage in order to prevent early osteoarthritis development, increase return-to-sport rate, and decrease healing time for OCD lesions. This chapter provides short but comprehensive to date knowledge about OCD on the knee of adolescents and young adults.

Keywords: osteochondritis dissecans, knee, adolescent, healing, OCD, JOCD

1. Introduction

Osteochondritis dissecans (OCD) of the knee is a pathological condition of subchondral bone resembling focal osteolysis with subsequent bone resorption, which may lead to osteochondral fragment separation. Several etiological concepts are presented for OCD development with the leading question of what was the first—bone or cartilage? This question was raised a couple of decades ago and was similar to that one about chicken and egg. The multifactorial theory that was presented accompanying different pathological pathways leads to the main pathology.

While plenty of studies existed describing the surgical treatment of OCD, different investigators presented their data about healing OCD lesions using conservative treatment or even "waitful watching" management with a healing rate of up to 67%. Despite such a good result, there are not any common practice guidelines for conservative treatment accepted by practitioners. OCD of the knee usually goes through several stages. The last one is the separation of osteochondral fragment, leaving a full-thickness osteochondral defect, which is usually filled with low-quality fibrocartilaginous tissue. This tissue provides a lesser extent of resistance to peak loading forces, which poses at risk subchondral bone, for further destruction and osteoarthritis development. This fact raises some questions about indications for surgical treatment, its timing, and best option for surgical management of OCD in a particular stage.

Knowing the fact that adolescents involved in competitive sports are usually predisposed to knee OCD—what management strategy would you apply to such patients? How would you choose the appropriate surgical method? Will you take to attention the stage and age of patient? When will you advise this patient to start sports activities? Which criteria would you use to decide about lesion healing? Is complete lesion healing possible after OCD? All these questions need to be summarized. This chapter provides short but comprehensive to date knowledge about OCD of the knee of adolescents and young adults.

2. Epidemiology

Two types of OCD in adolescents are established—juvenile and adult—depending on whether a growth plate of the distal femur is open or closed. Juvenile OCD of the knee has an incidence from 9.5 to 29 of 100,000 knees [1, 2]. There is a three times increased incidence in children after 12 years old in comparison with children 6–11 years old, and boys are affected around four times more frequently than girls [2]. Adolescents involved in professional sports represent a large cohort of patients affected by OCD [3]. Femoral condyles are commonly affected, and posterolateral aspect of medial condyle is the typical region of OCD location (77%) [4]. Less common regions are lateral condyle (17%), patella (7%), and tibial plateau (0.2%) [4]. Lesions are bilateral in 14–30% [5].

3. Etiology and pathology

Osteochondritis dissecans of the knee was first mentioned by König in 1888, who described focus of an inflammation of the bone cartilage interface. König supposed that direct and minimal trauma can result in isolated subchondral damage. Patients that did not have any trauma prior to symptoms development were assigned to "osteochondritis dissecans."

Many theories about OCD have been presented. It is well known that etiology-targeted treatment strategy is always the best. Thus, many investigators focused on looking for the main cause of the pathology. The pathology of OCD needs to be known to guide our way through its etiology.

According to pathological changes, OCD of the knee is usually divided into four stages, which may be seen in subchondral bone and adjoined articular cartilage [6]. Stage 1 is described as early subchondral osteopenia and usually is not detectable on X-ray, which remains a common way to visualize OCD lesions. Stage 2 represents bone marrow edema particularly located in subchondral bone. The bone is still viable in OCD lesions. Stage 3 is the most well-known stage by healthcare practitioners due to the possibility of X-ray to reveal radiolucency in subchondral bone representing its necrosis demarcated from healthy bone by sclerotic rim. Green and Banks were the first who discovered such necrosis and underlined intact articular cartilage adjoining OCD lesion (true stage 3) [7]. A variety of pathological changes was found by different investigators in OCD lesions on stage 3. Uozumi et al. found three types of bone morphology in OCD lesions—necrotic bone, viable ossifying trabecular bone, and absence of any bone. As the first type is inconsistent with the earliest study [7], other types rise the question of whether there are multiple morphological types of bone damage in OCD lesions or one process with consequent changing stages. For instance, Wagner described "malicious variant" with OCD lesions full of multiple bone fragments [8]. Other studies revealed the absence of any degenerative bone changes in stable OCD of the knee but the presence of fibrocartilaginous tissue on the periphery of the lesion between parents resembling that found between bone fragments in nonunion after bone fracture [9]—**Figure 1**.

Stage 4 usually occurs under continuing mechanical loading resulting in the loosening of the bone and cartilage followed by osteochondral fragment separation.

While most of the existing studies state that subchondral bone is to be damaged first, several pathways are described. According to the systematic review of Luca Andriolo et al., 28 articles present subchondral bone fracture as the starting point of pathology cascade, and eight articles state that ischemia is the first event followed by subchondral bone degeneration [10]. Thus, there are two main general theories: mechanical and vascular, followed by special biological, genetic, and endocrine factors, which may play role in OCD development.

The mainstay of the mechanical theory is collected data about relationship between chronic repetitive microtrauma, traumatic incidents, and consequent OCD development [11]. This theory has been supported by an epidemiological study, which revealed a relatively high proportion of adolescents involved in competitive sports activities [2]. Both acute and chronic repetitive trauma may result in subchondral fracture by themselves or in combination with other mechanical factors reported—discoid meniscus [12–14], tibial spine impingement [15], hypermobile anterior horn of meniscus [16], and joint instability and genu recurvatum [17]. Several metabolic conditions affect bone quality posing subchondral bone at risk for fracture—Wilson disease [18], hyper-IgE syndrome [19], low vitamin D3 level [20], and high human growth hormone level [21].

Other well-known theory is the vascular one. Adherents of this theory suppose that ischemia is the first event in subchondral bone followed by partial bone necrosis and subsequent fracture. The first histological confirmation of this theory is related with the study of Green & Banks, who found necrotic foci in the subchondral bone of femoral condyle [7]. Campbell and Ranawat later defined OCD as a focus of aseptic necrosis particularly developing in "locus minoris resistentiae" [22] of ossifying bone

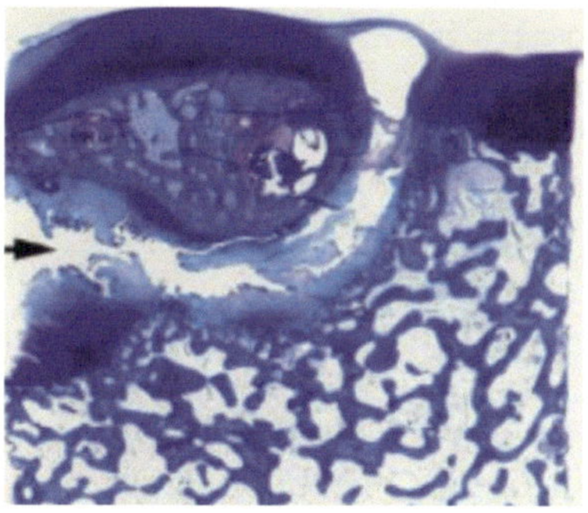

Figure 1.
Osteochondritis dissecans histology. Black arrow points to the fissure between maternal bone and osteochondral fragment. Note the presence of a sclerotic rim on maternal bone adjacent to the fissure and the presence of fibrous tissue precluding adequate union. From Bruns et al. [6].

of secondary ossification center in condylar epiphysis after repetitive microtrauma [23]. The ischemic nature of OCD lesions was advocated by Jans et al. Authors stated that terminal epiphyseal arteries do not have adequate collateral branches, resulting in abruption of subchondral bone vascular supply after minimal acute or chronic repetitive trauma [24]. The closed relationship between early epiphyseal vascular regression (up to 5 years old) and late enchondral ossification (up to 10 years old) of epiphyseal secondary ossification zones was described thoroughly by Ellerman et al. [25].

To date, pathophysiological pathway for OCD lesion development seems to be multifactorial: anatomy of epiphyseal vascular branches in zones of secondary enchondral ossification predisposes to subchondral bone fracture after minimal traumatic event, leading to bone necrosis, lack of cartilage supply, fissures emerging, and subsequent osteochondral fragment detachment.

4. History

History of OCD of the knee usually starts with pain, which can relate to previous traumatic episodes or not. The pain usually starts with prolonged physical activities, and worsens with deep squatting and load distribution to an affected leg [5]. As many patients with knee OCD are sportsmen, the main complaint is the inability to fully participate in competitions and even regular training activities. A separate type of history usually has patients sustained acute trauma after a period of prolonged knee pain. If such pain is long-lasting, it can be related with ongoing OCD of the knee, and the traumatic episode can lead to osteochondral fragment detachment. Such a patient may suffer from knee-locking episodes, popping, or knee catching. Cases of unstable OCD lesions are frequently accompanied by synovitis developing after osteochondral fragment partial detachment.

5. Physical examination

OCD of the knee in adolescents has poor clinical manifestation. In the case of stable OCD, there are not usually any positive provocative maneuvers. There is only one specific test described by Wilson—pain appears while tibia is internally rotated during knee extension from 30 to 90 degrees [26]. Pain alleviation, while tibia is externally rotated, is highly suspicious for OCD of femoral condyle in a typical location (posterolateral aspect of medial femoral condyle). In spite of relatively high specificity, this symptom has low clinical diagnostic value. Unstable OCD cases may be accompanied by knee effusion associated with smooth contours of the knee, positive patellar tap test, and restricted range of motion.

6. Imaging

Standing X-ray in three projections is a standard clinical protocol for OCD lesion evaluation. Anteroposterior, lateral, and notch-view usually are sufficient for diagnosis confirmation [27]. OCD lesion is usually described as either a crescent-shaped radiolucent area in subchondral bone or radiolucent line between bone fragment and parent bone with an area of sclerosis adjacent to radiolucent zone. In the case of unstable OCD with a detached osteochondral fragment, uneven contour of femoral condyle can be seen with an area of adjacent bone sclerosis. Despite the usefulness of radiography for diagnosis making, it is usually not possible to differentiate stable OCD lesions from unstable ones. So, radiography is of importance only as a first-contact diagnostic method.

MRI is the most informative method aiding in the visualization of all components of OCD lesions, including cartilage. T1 sequence is usually used for size measurement. T2 fat-saturated and PDFS sequences are used for bone marrow edema assessment, cartilage visualization, and most important for defining the type of OCD lesion according to its stability. De Smet et al. defined four MRI criteria of stability [28]:

1. A thin line of high-signal-intensity ≥5 mm in length at the interface between the lesion and underlying bone (fibrovascular granulation tissue);

2. A round area of homogeneous high-signal-intensity ≥5 mm in diameter beneath the lesion (cysts);

3. A focal defect with a width of ≥5 mm in the articular surface of the lesion (displacement of the lesion into the joint);

4. A high-signal-intensity line traversing articular cartilage into the lesion (articular fracture).

Despite relatively high sensitivity and specificity in adults, these criteria represented only 11% specificity in children [29]. After considering additional criteria by Kijowski et al., a specificity of 100% for children population achieved:

1. A high T2-signal-intensity rim or cysts surrounding an adult OCD lesion are unequivocal signs of instability

2. A high T2-signal-intensity rim surrounding a juvenile OCD lesion indicates instability only if it has the same signal intensity as adjacent joint fluid, is surrounded by a second outer rim of low T2-signal-intensity, or is accompanied by multiple breaks in the subchondral bone plate on T2-weighted MRI

3. Cysts surrounding a juvenile OCD lesion indicate instability only if they are multiple in number or large.

General visual characteristics of unstable and stable lesions described by Kijowski et al. are presented in **Figures 2** and **3**.

Defining the stability of OCD lesions is of utmost importance for guiding management. CT scan also takes an important part in OCD lesion visualization. It provides data about size and subchondral bone structure in detail and can aid in finding free osseous fragments in the knee joint [30]. CT scan has the possibility of fast and precise lesion assessment in both knees in case of two-sided knee OCD and serves as a good tool for finding accidental OCD lesions in the contralateral unaffected knee. Limitations include radiation exposure and the inability to assess cartilage status in OCD lesions. CT scan cannot define if the lesion is unstable or not.

Ultrasonography is rarely used in knee OCD imaging mainly because of its operator dependence and relatively low diagnostic accuracy [31].

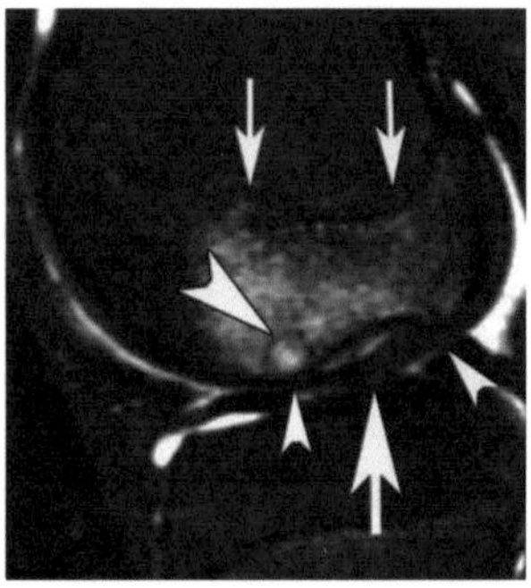

Figure 2.
Sagittal 1,5T fat suppressed T2w FSE MRI of the knee in a 15-year-old adolescent with confirmed unstable OCD lesion of the medial femoral condyle. OCD lesion consists of heterogeneous high- and low-signal-intensity (large arrow) areas and is surrounded by a single cyst of 6 mm in diameter (large arrowhead) and extensive bone marrow edema (small arrows). There is no disruption of the low-signal-intensity subchondral bone plate at edges of OCD lesion (small arrowheads). From: Kijowski et al. [28].

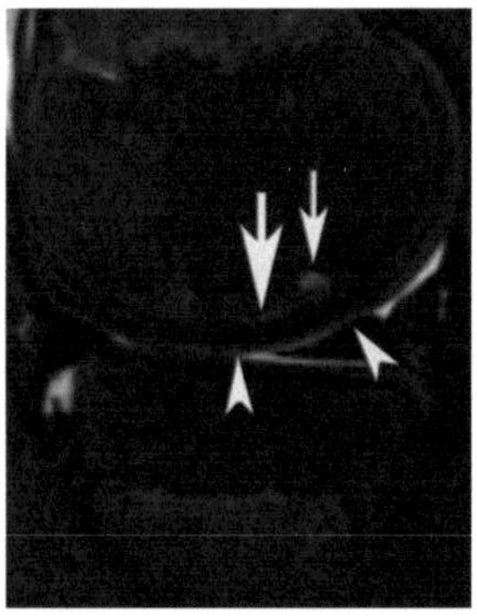

Figure 3.
Sagittal 1,5T fat suppressed T2w FSE MRI of the knee in a 12-year-old adolescent with confirmed stable OCD lesion of the medial femoral condyle. OCD lesion has uniform low-signal-intensity (large arrow) area that is surrounded by a single cyst 4 mm in diameter (small arrow). There is no disruption of low-signal-intensity subchondral bone plate at the edges of OCD lesion (arrowheads). From: Kijowski et al. [29].

Bone scintigraphy is a method that is possible to provide data about bone perfusion of an OCD lesion. Almost absolutely lacking specificity in defining different stages of OCD, this imaging modality is rather a historical one. Nowadays 3-T MRI method of "arterial spin labeling" was developed to assess perfusion in femoral condyles similarly to scintigraphy [32].

7. Classifications

There are plenty of classifications described nowadays for knee OCD. A few of them are useful in treatment strategy choosing. As radiography and CT scan cannot accurately describe lesions' stability, most investigators attempted to find the best MRI classification either for treatment strategy defining or for preoperative planning. The most important among MRI classifications are the aforementioned classification by De Smet et al.'s and Kijowski et al.'s modifications for lesion stability assessment [28, 29, 33].

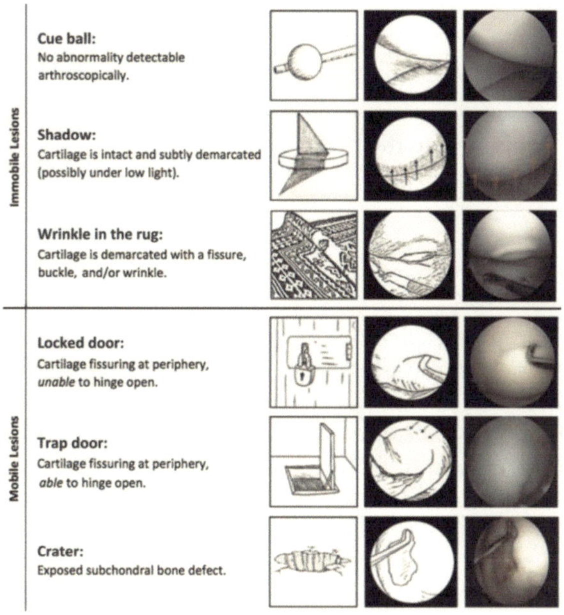

Figure 4.
ROCK study group arthroscopic OCD lesion classification. Six stages were described with 1–3 being stable and 4–6 unstable.

Arthroscopy remains to be a gold standard for the assessment of OCD lesion stability [1]. Various classifications are described. Most of them consist of four stages [34–36], where third stage is an unstable OCD lesion with a partially detached osteochondral fragment and fourth stage is a completely detached fragment with a free intraarticular body. To days, a new classification was developed by the ROCK study group consisting of six stages based on arthroscopic lesion appearance (**Figure 4**).

8. Treatment strategy

There are two main options—conservative and surgical treatments. As OCD of the knee is progressing disease, the main goal of treatment of unstable lesions is to prevent their destabilization and achieve full lesion healing.

Healing of some OCD lesions reaches 50–67% in 6–12 months [5, 37, 38]. Despite such good results, the current literature volume accumulated has scarce data about different conservative treatment methods with moderate quality studies mostly due to the inability to correct allocation of patients and non-randomized study designs [11].

In a recent systematic review, Andriolo et al. found 24 case-series studies and three case reports for conservative treatment of OCD lesions. Only 12 studies had one treatment method such as immobilization, physical instrumental therapy, or physical activity restriction. Fourteen studies describe combinations of conservative methods of treatment. Overall healing was 61.4% ranging from 10.4% to 95.8% [11]. Despite such heterogeneous data, negative prognostic values for healing were also described:

1. Lesion size (large size correlated with low overall healing rate)

2. Severe lesion stages based on different classifications

3. Older age

4. Combination with discoid meniscus

5. Long period from onset to the first consultation

6. Mechanical symptoms

7. Atypical lesion location (lateral femoral condyle, patella, and tibial condyles)

While some studies report 80–90% healing rate of stable OCD lesions, using physical activity restriction and quadriceps muscle strengthening [39], others report only 30% healing rate and 67% as "no changes" [40]. Such differences may have been appeared due to maturity status or other abovementioned factors confounding. To minimize influence of confounding factors on the healing rate, Krause et al. developed a nomogram for probability of healing assessment [38]. He used multivariate analysis of independent factors on 37 OCD lesions and found three independent factors: age, cyst-like lesion normalized width, and overall lesion normalized width—0–10 points, for each of assessing factors. The overall score is linked with probability scale (**Figure 5**—the example).

Generally, stable OCD lesions followed every 3 months with different authors suggesting either 3 or 6 months of conservative treatment prior to surgery referral decision-making [5, 11, 41].

Despite good short-term results of conservative treatment for juvenile stable OCD lesions, a recent study by Sanders et al. described bothering long-term results—in up to 30% of patients treated nonoperatively osteoarthritis was developed at 35 years [42]. Another long-term study by the same author reports osteoarthritis development cumulative incidence of 70% at 30 years after osteochondral fragment excision in patients with the last stage of knee OCD and 51% incidence in patients at 30 years

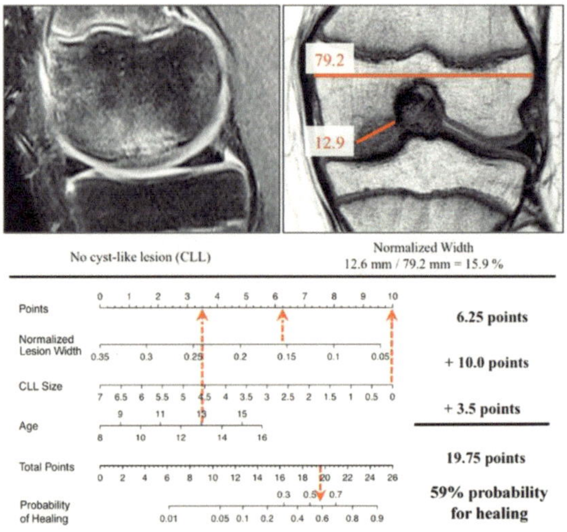

Figure 5.
Prediction of healing probability after 6 months of nonoperative treatment based on normalized lesion width, cyst-like lesion (CLL) size, and patient age. The case is a 13-year-old patient, who showed a tendency toward healing after 6 months and showed complete healing in 12 months. From: Krause et al. [38].

after osteochondral fragment preservation [43]. This relatively high incidence determines the need for thorough timing of operative treatment.

As large part of patients with OCD of the knee is represented by professional sportsmen, the time of OCD lesion healing really matters. Faster lesion healed—faster weight-bearing activities may be achieved, and shorter return-to-sport can be reached.

In summary, indications for operative treatment of the knee OCD in adolescents are as follows:

1. Signs of instability defined by Kijowski et al. on MRI. Elective surgery may be planned but patient must observe a special regimen of non-weight bearing and activity restriction.

2. Mechanical symptoms emergence in addition to preoperative imaging data about osteochondral fragment separation. Surgery needs to be provided as fast as possible to capture a chance of osteochondral fragment refixation.

3. More than 3 months of conservative treatment without any healing signs.

9. Operative treatment

The type of surgical intervention in adolescent knee OCD depends on several factors: stability and size of the lesion and presence or absence of mechanical symptoms in patient.

Surgical treatment usually starts from arthroscopy of the knee. Infrapatellar plica, medial plica, and partial Hoffa pad resection are necessary for better visualization of condylar cartilage. The main goal is to correctly assess if the OCD lesion is stable or not. Visually stable JOCD may be represented by fully intact cartilage either without any color changes or may have dim color compared to neighboring regions of intact cartilage. Cartilage above the lesion may be depressed or fissured on the periphery of the lesion or can be partially detached. Villous overlays may be seen in patients with partially fissured cartilage.

9.1 Stable OCD lesions

When the lesion is stable, there is usually fibrocartilaginous layer between osteochondral fragment and maternal bone, resembling tissue that is usually can be found in pseudarthroses between bone fragments [9]. This finding supports data about failed ossification as the main barrier for OCD lesion to heal [44]. So far, local stimulation of osteogenesis is the main goal of OCD lesion treatment. It can be either mechanical stimulation or biological.

Common mechanical stimulation of bone regeneration in stable OCD lesions is drilling [1, 5]. There are two types of drilling: antegrade (retroarticular) and retrograde (transarticular or transchondral). Retroarticular drilling has the advantage of cartilage preservation but method is not universal and depends on OCD lesion location [45]. For instance, if OCD lesion is located posteriorly in condyle or in the center of the weight-bearing surface of cartilage, it is possible to reach this zone from the lateral subphyseal area of condyle, used as starting point for drilling. The use of fluoroscopy guidance during retroarticular drilling is associated with radiation exposure.

Anteriorly located lesions are difficult to be drilled from this position. Transarticular drilling is faster, and there is no need for fluoroscopy guidance because drilling is performed under direct visual control by an arthroscope. Nonetheless, transarticular drilling is associated with cartilage damage. Cartilage appearance may have changed for years after transarticular drilling as advocated [46]. Otherwise, long-term studies with well-done designs are needed to advocate if transarticular drilling has a negative effect on knee functioning or early osteoarthritis development.

Gunton et al. published a thorough systematic review of studies that investigated either transarticular or retrograde drilling of OCD lesions [45]. Despite meta-analysis was not possible to carry out and the high heterogeneity of studies, the authors found no significant differences according to lesion healing effectiveness. There was 86% healing rate for retroarticular drilling and 91% for transarticular. Patient-reported outcomes were also comparable. Time to heal was lower in lesions after transarticular drilling (4–5 months) compared to retroarticular (5–6 months). Despite that facts, 36.9% lateral condyles were drilled in retroarticular group compared with 5.3% in transarticular, for healing rate comparison,48% and 6.3%—for time-to-heal comparing, respectively. Knowing that many factors affect the healing rate in OCD lesions, including lesion location, the results must be interpreted with caution.

The authors of this chapter carried out their own systematic review for OCD lesion drilling in children aged before 18 years old, only nine full-text studies were included in the analysis. We found 95.3% cumulative healing rate of OCD lesions after retrograde drilling and 76.8% after transarticular drilling [47]. Because of such heterogeneous information represented across the literature, there is no evidence of which type of drilling is preferable currently considering either healing rate or time-to-heal.

9.2 Unstable OCD lesions

Unstable lesions may be represented as partially or completely detached osteochondral fragments. Osteochondral fragment detached from their place and becomes incongruent with time, so there is a need for urgent treatment of patients with unstable OCD lesions suspected in MRI. If we have a deal with unstable but partially detached fragment, fixation of the fragment is the most valuable option. It can be carried out by metal screws, absorbable pins, Kirshner wires, or even autologous bone sticks [48]. A recent systematic review carried out by Leland et al. reported 67–100% healing rate after osteochondral fragment fixation in skeletally matured knees. No significant differences were found in context with healing rate between types of fixator, and complications included reoperations for cartilage resurfacing, loose body removal, or unplanned hardware removal [48]. Kocher et al. found 84,6% radiographic healing rate in adolescent OCD using fragment fixation independently of device used for fixation [49]. Adachi et al. reported 77% healing rate after osteochondral fragment fixation using bioabsorbable pins [50]. Wu et al. found 76% healing rate in both skeletally immature and mature knees in their multicenter study. They reported no differences between mature and immature knees in the context of healing rate [51].

9.3 Full-thickness cartilage lesions in the last stage of OCD

There is a high rate of osteoarthritis development after osteochondral fragment detachment—a cumulative incidence of 70% at 30 years was reported recently. Moreover, the cumulative incidence of arthroplasty is 32% at 30 years [43]. To avoid these complications and to achieve a good quality of life for patients with osteochondral defects different methods exist.

For lesions less than 2 cm^2, microfracture procedure proved to be the first-line treatment method [52]. Damaging subchondral bone with special awl results in multipotent stromal cell effluxes followed by fibrocartilage filling the defect. It provides good short-term results in context with patient-related outcomes [53]. Despite relatively good short-term results after microfracture procedure, there is an incidence of 45% for knee replacement at median of 12 years after this procedure [54]. Hyaline cartilage predominantly contains collagen type 2 while fibrocartilage, which fills osteochondral defects after microfracture, mainly consists of collagen type 1 [55]. Therefore, fibrocartilage does not have properties of normal hyaline articular cartilage and cannot withstand weight-bearing loads as well as intact articular hyaline cartilage [56]. Despite being the first-line treatment for osteochondral defects smaller than 2 cm^2, recent systematic review reported increased fill of the defect while using deep drilling comparative with microfracturing. Free access to bone marrow space can be achieved using deep drilling, while fractured bone with osteocyte necrosis was found after microfracture procedure [57]. Two studies reported superior cartilage restoration while implementing deep drilling (6 mm depth) instead of microfracture procedure [58, 59].

Osteochondral autologous transplantation (OAT) or mosaicplasty is another option to fill the full-thickness osteochondral defect. Osteochondral plugs from non-weight bearing region of femoral condyles are harvested and transferred to osteochondral defect in this method. Mosaicplasty has good mid-term and long-term results in the context of activity, and patient outcome scores risk of failure in patients with osteochondral lesions sized more than 3 cm^2 [60, 61]. Pareek et al. recognized in their meta-analysis that microfracture has 2.4 times more risk of failure compared with mosaicplasty [60]. Gudas et al. found a 21-times higher risk of failure after microfracture procedure compared with OAT in patients with full-thickness lesions of more than 3 cm^2 only after OCD [62]. Solheim et al. also reported noticeably increased patient-reported outcomes after mosaicplasty compared with microfracture procedure at long-term follow-up [63]. OAT has several complications, including cartilage hypertrophy, at the periphery of osteochondral defect and donor site morbidity while using more than two osteochondral plugs [64]. That limits the implementation of OAT in adolescents involved in professional sports activities. Limitations can be partially avoided using allograft-OAT called in literature OCA (osteochondral allograft transplantation). This technique allows for more thorough graft matching with the defect and, therefore, may be used in cartilage defects more than 4 cm^2 [52].

Autologous chondrocyte implantation (ACI) and its 3rd generation—matrix-induced autologous chondrocyte implantation (MACI)—are promising techniques for cartilage restoration in patients with osteochondral defects more than 2 cm^2 [52]. The main feature associated with MACI is the need for two operations to be performed. This fact significantly affects the rehabilitation period and return to sport velocity. The main goal of first operation is to harvest cartilage from non-weight bearing zones, usually intercondylar notch. After that, 6-week production period is needed for colony of MSC to grow and colony formation. Seeded on a special porcine collagen membrane, MSC is attached to osteochondral defect. MACI is superior to microfracture procedure in patients that have more than 2 cm^2 cartilage lesions at 2-year [65] and 5-year follow-up [66], according to results of patient-reported outcome measures.

Autologous induced matrix chondrogenesis (AMIC) is another technology, the main peculiarity of which is absence of second operation necessity. After lesion site debridement and subchondral bone exposure drilling perform followed by the application of ready-to-use collagen I/III membrane supported by fibrin glue [67]. Efflux of MSC from bone marrow of condyle and its proliferation and differentiation in special microenvironment provide cartilage restoration and hyaline-like tissue formation [68]. Several studies support the supremacy of AMIC over microfracture procedures in osteochondral defects more than 2 cm^2 on context with both patient-reported outcomes and MRI data achieved [67–69].

Another promising method for one-stage cartilage restoration is minced cartilage preparation and usage. Basic science for this method was represented by several authors [70–73] and a few clinical studies conducted to date [74]. Salzmann et al. figured out that chondrocytes in live cartilage after slicing induce their proliferation and differentiation, produce intercellular matrix, and have the ability to fill cartilage defects [70]. It was also found that the smaller cartilage particles are—the bigger amount of ECM is going to be produced after cartilage slicing [73] and more efficient chondrocytes outgrowth is Ref. [75]. Firstly, reported by Albrecht et al., particulate autologous cartilage implantation (or minced cartilage implantation) procedure proved the clinical efficacy of cartilage autograft implantation system (CAIS) in the study of cole BJ et al., who reported marked improvement with statistically significant differences for KOOS and IKDC scores in favor of CAIS compared with microfracture procedure [76]. The surgical technique includes harvesting cartilage from non-weight bearing part of condylar cartilage (usually in the region of intercondylar notch), processing of cartilage (cartilage fragmentation with a shaver or other devices), cartilage defect preparation (defect walls debridement and removing of calcified layer), minced cartilage paste preparation using either fibrin glue or different orthobiologic substances—BMAC, PRP, and PRF [74, 77].

A few clinical studies confirmed positive results of minced cartilage implantation procedures. Christensen et al. reported markedly improved MOCART-MRI score, patient-reported outcomes, and more than 80% bone defect filling at 1 year after operation in eight patients using a combination of autologous bone graft and autologous cartilage chips technique supported by fibrin glue. All patients had osteochondral defects developed as the last stage of OCD [78]. Massen et al. revealed statistically significant improvement in functional knee score and MOCART score at 2 years, after minced cartilage implantation in 27 patients, and concluded that minced cartilage technique can be a good alternative to currently existing ACI/MACI techniques [79]. Cugat et al. reported excellent clinical, MRI, and patient-reported functional outcomes in 15 patients at 15 months after minced cartilage technique implementation with platelet-rich and platelet-poor 50/50 plasma addition [80].

Particulated juvenile allograft cartilage (PJAC) is the technology resembling minced cartilage procedure. The main difference is that PJAC represented by juvenile hyaline cartilage consisted of immature chondrocytes that provide increased proliferative and metabolic activity, obtained from donors, and has 45 days to be viable after the cells package [81, 82], while there are no clinical studies for use of PJAC currently available [52]. However, Ao et al. found more hyaline-like cartilage content at 1 month and 3 months after cartilage chips implantation in minipigs compared with PJAC implantation with no significant differences at 6 months [83].

10. Biological stimulation in OCD treatment

Biological stimulation is another way to improve bone regeneration locally. Orthobiological products, such as platelet-rich plasma (PRP) and bone marrow aspirate concentrate (BMAC), contain different growth factors, improving cell proliferation, migration, and differentiation [84–86]. BMAC also has multipotent stem cells, which can differentiate into different lineages themselves taking part in tissue restoration [87]. There is a literature gap about biological preparations implementation in complex surgical treatment of knee OCD.

Sharma et al. reported six adult OCD unstable ICRS and three lesions completely healed in 4 months using fragment fixation with metal compression screws and adjuvant intraarticular PRP injection treatment. The authors' technique was represented by three intraarticular injections of PRP every 3 weeks starting on 12 postoperative days, and 8–10 ml PRP was used for each injection [88]. Davidson et al. shared the results of 52 stable juvenile OCD lesions treatment with an average size of 4.07 cm^2 by retroarticular drilling and BMAC augmentation back-filling through pin channel. 76.9% of lesions were healed at a mean of 10.6 months [89]. Later Andelman et al. described a technique for retroarticular core decompression of stable OCD lesions by retroarticular over drilling of femoral condyle using a drill bit with subsequent curette OCD lesion decompression and implementing BMAC-DBM paste [90]. No results have yet been published to analyze this treatment method. Baldassarri et al. recently reported good results using bone marrow-derived cell transplantation technique for restoration of osteochondral defects [91]. The technique implies a collagen scaffold, embedded with concentrated bone marrow aspirate and platelet-rich gel. Authors found significantly better Tegner and IKDC scores at 1 year after the operation and 75–100% lesion filling on MRI-MOCART score in 13 out of 18 patients. De Girolamo et al. noted lower VAS scores in patients undergone AMIC procedure with BMAC augmentation compared with AMIC procedure alone for full-thickness osteochondral defects, with significant difference in Lysholm score at 6 and 12 months after operation in favor of AMIC with BMAC procedure [68]. This finding is important in the context of the rehabilitation period shortening and faster return to sport.

Retroarticular drilling with PRP intralesional injections technique is currently used in N.F. Filatov Children's City Hospital of Moscow Healthcare Ministry by prof. Vybornov D. Yu. et al. This method was developed for stable OCD lesions and implies retroarticular drilling of the lesion with combined fluoroscopy and arthroscopy assistance—3 or 4 drill holes made—with subsequent slow (2 minutes long) PRP injection through the drill channel using 20G long needle and 3-minute exposition before needle withdrawal (**Figure 6**). PRP is derived from peripheral blood after 2-stage centrifugation according to the platelet-safe, Bausset et al. technique previously described maximizing live platelet count in the final product [92].

A 13-year-old adolescent was admitted to orthopedics and traumatology department of N.F. Filatov Children's City Hospital of Moscow Healthcare Ministry with 9-month long complaints of knee pain that were worsening after physical activities and deep squatting. Knee provocative tests were negative. MRI and CT scan revealed an OCD lesion in medial femoral condyle without instability signs (**Figure 7A** and **D**). The patient undergone retroarticular drilling and PRP intralesional injection procedure. Touch-down weight-bearing started 1 month after the operation. A 2-month follow-up MRI revealed partial lesion healing (**Figure 7B**) and a 6-month MRI and CT scan showed restoration of subchondral bone without any signs of cartilage pathology (**Figure 7C** and **E**).

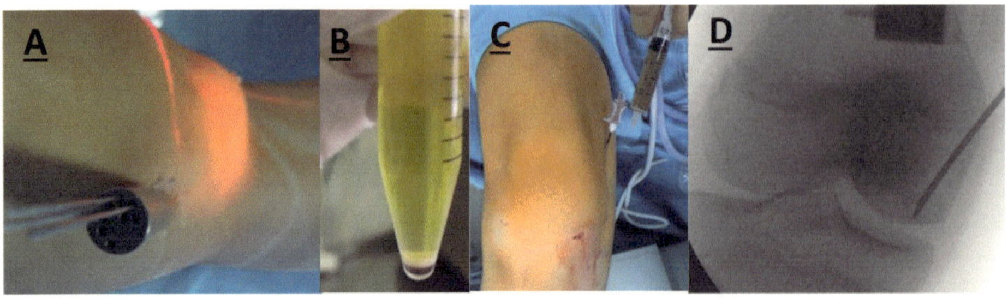

Figure 6
(A–D). Retroarticular drilling with PRP intralesional injection technique. OCD lesion is over drilled from starting point of approximately 0,5 cm under the growth plate under fluoroscopy control (A). PRP is prepared 30 minutes before operation with Bausset et al.'s protocol (B). PRP is slowly injected inside the lesion (C). Fluoroscopy control of needle position is mandatory before PRP injection (D).

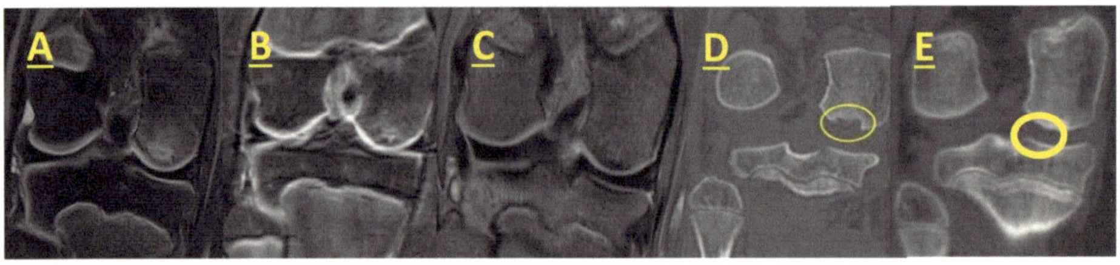

Figure 7
(A—E). A 13-year-old patient with a stable OCD lesion was revealed on MRI (A) and CT scan (D). Bone marrow high-intensity-signal on PDFS MRI without any signs of instability, and the low-intensity line between progeny and parent bone can be found representing ossification impairment (A). The subchondral bone defect is shown on CT scan (D). Retroarticular drilling and PRP intralesional injection procedure were performed. The 2-month follow-up frontal PDFS MRI revealed relatively low bone marrow signal intensity (B). Moreover, the low-intensity line became shorter representing bone restoration process (B). Frontal PDFS MRI and CT scan at 6 months after the operation showed almost full subchondral bone restoration (E) and intact cartilage with minimal residual changes in subchondral bone (D).

This method was assessed in a comparative study that is yet unpublished. Fifty-five patients with femoral condylar OCD were included in the study and divided into three groups based on treatment method—retroarticular drilling and intralesional PRP injection, transarticular drilling without any additives, or transarticular drilling with intraarticular PRP injection. In total, 12 out of 15 OCD lesions in the retroarticular drilling+PRP group healed completely and three patients with shallow but wide and long OCD lesions did not have signs of healing at a median 10-month follow-up. Despite no statistically significant differences in OCD lesion size between groups were found, PRP implementation led to decreased time-to-heal: 6 months for complete healing in PRP groups versus median 10 months in the no-PRP group. We suggest retroarticular drilling with PRP intralesional injections for deep and short stable OCD lesions.

11. Defining healing of OCD lesion

To days, treatment guidelines for OCD of the knee are lacking evidence. One of the reasons is the lack of commonly adopted healing criteria and the absence of correlation between symptoms and OCD stage except stage 4 when mechanical symptoms usually guide the diagnosis [93]. Parikh et al. reported low interrater reliability

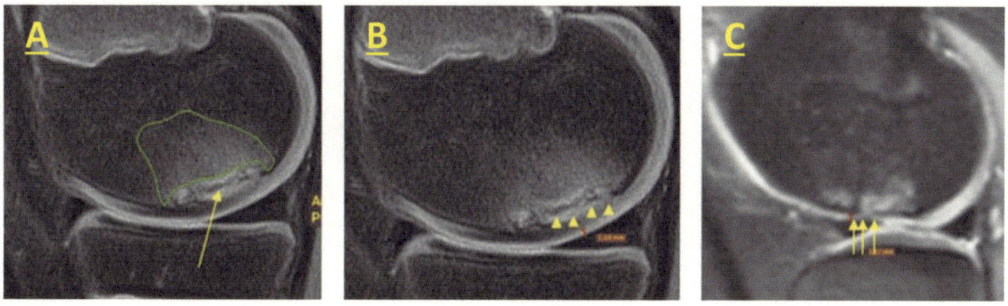

Figure 8.
Four main parameters are assessed to calculate general healing. The bone substance edema (circled with a continuous line—A), the degree of consolidation (the line between the osteochondral fragment of the lesion and the maternal bone is indicated by an arrow in Figure A), bone structure (estimated by density and structure of the bone tissue—B), and articular cartilage structure (indicated by arrows in Figure C).

for radiographic assessment of healing at 6 months after operation [94]. Wall et al. developed a reliable radiographic method of OCD lesion healing assessment based on a subjective assessment of five parameters on a continuous slider scale from −100 to +100 points [93]. Radiographic features assessed included articular surface shape, boundary, sclerosis, ossification, lesion size, and overall healing. Authors reported substantial to excellent interrater reliability at 2–24 months with ICC values from 0.77 to 0.88 [93]. This reliable method is perfectly fit for the assessment of OCD lesion healing independent from place of residence. Limitations include radiation exposure and inability to visualize cartilage.

Based on the study by Wall et al. [93] group of specialists in pediatric sports medicine and musculoskeletal radiologist of N.F. Filatov Children's City Hospital of Moscow Healthcare Ministry and the department of pediatric surgery of Russian National Research Medical University made an adaption of the abovementioned scale for MRI [95]. An expert group was conformed consisting of a 6-year medical university student, three 2nd-year residents, one pediatric orthopedic surgeon, and one musculoskeletal radiologist. After two rounds of learning by PowerPoint presentation for scale assessment rules, 34 knee PDFS MRI was assessed at different time points before and after operation. Five MRI-based features were determined (**Figure 8**): the degree of bone edema (**Figure 8A**), fragment consolidation (**Figure 8A**), subchondral bone structure (**Figure 8B**), articular cartilage damage (**Figure 8C**), and general lesion healing. Unlike the original Wall et al.'s study, general healing was calculated as a mean of four previous features assessed by experts. Excellent reliability was found for all parameters with ICC values of 0.97–0,99 except the degree of bone marrow edema on the latest follow-up MRI—0.54.

A comparative study on the treatment of stable OCD lesions is currently on go using this novel MRI healing score for OCD of femoral condyles.

12. Authors' preferred strategy for adolescent OCD of the knee management

While most of the adolescent patients with knee OCD are active and 53% of them are involved in competitive sports activities according to statistics from the department of orthopedics and traumatology of N.F. Filatov Children's City Hospital of Moscow Healthcare Ministry, not only 100% healing rate but also as fast as possible

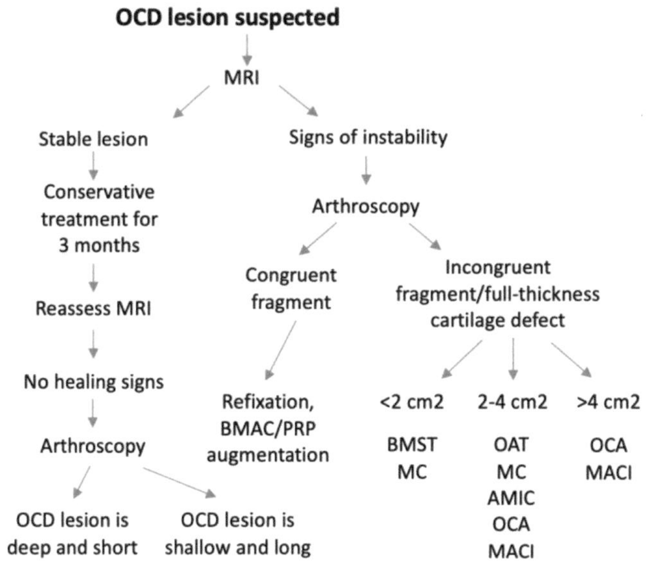

Figure 9.
Authors' preferred algorithm of OCD treatment in adolescents. BMST—bone marrow stimulation techniques, MC—minced cartilage technique, OAT—osteochondral autograft transplantation, AMIC—autologous matrix-induced chondrogenesis, OCA—osteochondral allograft implantation, and MACI—matrix-induced autologous chondrocyte implantation.

return to the abovementioned activities is awaited by patients. Appropriate treatment usually starts with appropriate history taking and imaging. We use several obligate questions for all patients about which mechanical symptoms they have, the longevity of their complaints, and prior treatment attempts. The presence of mechanical symptoms or knee effusion episodes always makes us suppose an unstable OCD lesion. MRI usually assists in lesion-type clarification. In the case of stable OCD lesions, conservative treatment usually starts, including affected limb unbearing, physical therapy without weight-bearing exercises, pulsed electromagnetic fields application, massage, and laser therapy. MRI is reassessed at 3 months. If no healing signs are presented—elective surgery is indicated. Stable OCD lesions are managed either by transchondral drilling with one intraarticular PRP injection after joint drying or with retroarticular drilling with intralesional PRP injection. Note that long and shallow OCD lesions are not fit well for retroarticular drilling techniques because of the risk of not reaching all zones of OCD lesions, which can later lead to lesion persistence.

Unstable OCD lesions are managed by refixation using metal screws either with compression cancellous screw or with headless screw. We prefer cancellous metal compression screw for large osteochondral fragments to achieve good compression forces at the progeny-perant bone line. For small fragments headless screws are appropriate for use because of the risk of progeny bone fragmentation.

Full-thickness defects management depends on the defect's size. Small defects less than 2 cm^2 usually undergo bone marrow stimulation (BMS) procedures. We prefer 1.5-mm pin drilling to a depth of no less than 1-cm and 5-mm distance between drill holes. Intraarticular PRP injection is routinely used in our department after each BMS procedure. For 2–4 cm^2-sized lesions osteochondral autograft transplantation (OAT), minced cartilage (MC) with fibrin glue and BMAC implementation, autologous matrix-induced chondrogenesis (AMIC), osteochondral allograft implantation (OCA), and matrix-induced autologous chondrocyte implantation (MACI) preferable depending on its availability for patient. For those defects whose size is more than 4 cm^2, OCA and MACI are the only methods that have evidence in the context of safety and possibility for use.

Brief authors' preferred algorithm for OCD treatment in adolescents is presented in **Figure 9**.

13. Conclusion

Osteochondritis dissecans of the knee in adolescents is potentially harmful disease, which mostly affects active children after 12 years old, usually involved in sports activities [5]. OCD generally has four stages with the last one representing osteochondral separation [6], potentially leading to early osteoarthritis and knee replacement if not managed appropriately [43, 96]. Proper OCD imaging allows to define stability of the lesion, which is a guide for treatment [97].

Stable lesions can be treated conservatively using several methods, evidence for which is not clear yet [11]. Conservative treatment can last from 3 to 6 months, and healing signs lacking at 6 months is an indication for surgery. Arthroscopy-assisted drilling for subchondral bone reparation improvement is the gold standard for stable lesions treatment regardless of the type [45, 98–101]. Biological stimulation procedures are generally safe and proven to decrease healing time and increase the healing rate for nonunion [102–105]. PRP or BMAC potentially can be applied in OCD cases [88, 89].

The goal of fourth stage OCD treatment is to deal with osteochondral defects. Depending on its size different options are available nowadays [34, 52, 53, 70, 72, 106–113]. Bone marrow stimulation techniques (BMST), minced cartilage implantation (MC), or autologous induced chondrogenesis (AMIC) with membranes for lesions less than 2 cm^2 are followed by osteochondral autograft transplantation (OAT), osteochondral allograft transplantation (OCA), matrix-induced autologous chondrocyte transplantation (MACI), or minced cartilage implantation (MC) in lesions 2–4 cm^2. Defects more than 4 cm^2 require OCA or MACI for getting better outcome [52].

All methods have different cost-efficiency, availability, and complications. The individual decision must be taken for each patient considering all influencing factors.

Acknowledgements

We would like to acknowledge coworkers of N.F. Filatov Children's City Hospital of Moscow Healthcare Ministry, department of pediatric orthopedics and traumatology: Nataliya Trusova, Ekaterina Kardash.

Conflict of interest

The authors declare no conflict of interest.

Special thanks

We would like to address special thanks to contributors of our surgical operations, coworkers of the N.F. Filatov Children's City Hospital of Moscow Healthcare Ministry:

transfusiology department head—Marina Khlebnikova; Anesthesiologists—Alexander Leshkevitch, Anna Shaginyan; operation nurses—Darya Panfilova, Nataliya Kiyayeva, Lyudmila Klyueva, Tatiana Kotova; and residents of pediatric surgery department of Russian National Research Medical University.

Author details

Andrey Semenov[1*], Dmitriy Vybornov[1], Nikolaj Tarasov[2], Vladimir Krestyashin[1], Ivan Isaev[2] and Vladimir Koroteev[2]

1 Russian National Research Medical University, Moscow, Russian Federation

2 N.F. Filatov Children's City Hospital of Moscow Healthcare Ministry, Moscow, Russian Federation

*Address all correspondence to: dru4elos@gmail.com

References

[1] Chau MM, Klimstra MA, Wise KL, Ellermann JM, Tóth F, Carlson CS, et al. Osteochondritis Dissecans: Current understanding of epidemiology, etiology, management, and outcomes. The Journal of Bone and Joint Surgery. American Volume. 2021;**103**(12):1132-1151

[2] Kessler JI, Nikizad H, Shea KG, Jacobs JC, Bebchuk JD, Weiss JM. The demographics and epidemiology of osteochondritis dissecans of the knee in children and adolescents. The American Journal of Sports Medicine. 2014;**42**(2):320-326

[3] Kocher MS, Tucker R, Ganley TJ, Flynn JM. Management of osteochondritis dissecans of the knee: Current concepts review. The American Journal of Sports Medicine. 2006;**34**(7):1181-1191

[4] Hefti F, Beguiristain J, Krauspe R, Möller-Madsen B, Riccio V, Tschauner C, et al. Osteochondritis dissecans: A multicenter study of the European Pediatric Orthopedic Society. Journal of Pediatric Orthopedic Society. 1999;**8**(4):231-245

[5] Masquijo J, Kothari A. Juvenile osteochondritis dissecans (JOCD) of the knee: Current concepts review. EFORT Open Review. 2019;**4**(5):201-212

[6] Bruns J, Werner M, Habermann C. Osteochondritis Dissecans: Etiology, pathology, and imaging with a special focus on the knee joint. Cartilage. 2018;**9**(4):346-362

[7] Green WT, Banks HH. Osteochondritis dissecans in children. The Journal of Bone and Joint Surgery. American Volume. 1953;**35**(1):26-47

[8] Wagner H. Surgical treatment of osteochondritis dissecans, a cause of arthritis deformans of the knee. Rev Chir Orthop Reparatrice Appar Mot. 2022;**50**:335-352

[9] Yonetani Y, Nakamura N, Natsuume T, Shiozaki Y, Tanaka Y, Horibe S. Histological evaluation of juvenile osteochondritis dissecans of the knee: A case series. Knee Surgery, Sports Traumatology, Arthroscopy. 2010;**18**(6):723-730

[10] Andriolo L, Crawford DC, Reale D, Zaffagnini S, Candrian C, Cavicchioli A, et al. Osteochondritis Dissecans of the knee: Etiology and pathogenetic mechanisms. A systematic review. Cartilage. 2018;**11**(3):273-290

[11] Andriolo L, Candrian C, Papio T, Cavicchioli A, Perdisa F, Filardo G. Osteochondritis Dissecans of the knee - Conservative treatment strategies: A systematic review. Cartilag. 2019;**10**

[12] Ishikawa M, Adachi N, Nakamae A, Deie M, Ochi M. Progression of stable juvenile osteochondritis dissecans after 10 years of meniscectomy of the discoid lateral meniscus. Journal of Pediatric Orthopaedics Part B. 2017;**26**(5):487-490

[13] Deie M, Ochi M, Sumen Y, Kawasaki K, Adachi N, Yasunaga Y, et al. Relationship between osteochondritis dissecans of the lateral femoral condyle and lateral menisci types. Journal of Pediatric Orthopedic. 2006;**26**(1):79-82

[14] Kamei G, Adachi N, Deie M, Nakamae A, Nakasa T, Shibuya H, et al. Characteristic shape of the lateral femoral condyle in patients with

osteochondritis dissecans accompanied by a discoid lateral meniscus. Journal of Orthopaedic Science. 2012;**17**(2):124-128

[15] Bramer JAM, Maas M, Dallinga RJ, te Slaa RL, Vergroesen DA. Increased external tibial torsion and osteochondritis dissecans of the knee. Clinical Orthopaedics and Related Research. 2004;**422**:175-179

[16] Camathias C, Hirschmann MT, Vavken P, Rutz E, Brunner R, Gaston MS. Meniscal suturing versus screw fixation for treatment of osteochondritis dissecans: Clinical and magnetic resonance imaging results. Arthroscopy: The Journal of Arthroscopic and Related Surgery. 2014;**30**(10):1269-1279

[17] Crawford DC, Safran MR. Osteochondritis dissecans of the knee. Journal of the American Academy of Orthopaedic Surgeons. 2006;**14**:90-100

[18] Park NH, Kim HS, Yi SY, Min BC. Multiple osteochondritis dissecans of knee joint in a patient with Wilson disease, focusing on magnetic resonance findings. Knee Surgical Related Research. 2013;**25**(4):225-229

[19] Kiliç SS, Sanal O, Tezcan I, Ersoy F. Osteochondritis dissecans in a patient with hyperimmunoglobulin E syndrome. The Turkish Journal of Pediatrics. 2002;**44**(4):357-359

[20] Bruns J, Werner M, Soyka M. Is vitamin D insufficiency or deficiency related to the development of osteochondritis dissecans? Knee Surgery, Sports Traumatology, Arthroscopy. 2016;**24**(5):1575-1579

[21] Hussain WM, Hussain HM, Hussain MS, Ho SSW. Human growth hormone and the development of osteochondritis dissecans lesions. Knee Surgery, Sports Traumatology, Arthroscopy. 2011;**19**(12):2108-2110

[22] Ribbing S. The hereditary multiple epiphyseal disturbance and its consequences for the Aetiogenesis of Locai, Malacjas-Particularly the Osteochondrosis Dissecans. Acta Orthopedic. 1954;**24**(1-4):286-299

[23] Campbell CJ, Ranawat CS. Osteochondritis dissecans: The question of etiology. The Journal of Trauma. 1966;**6**(2):201-221

[24] Jans L, Jaremko J, Ditchfield M, de Coninck T, Huysse W, Moon A, et al. Ossification variants of the femoral condyles are not associated with osteochondritis dissecans. European Journal of Radiology. 2012;**81**(11):3384-3389

[25] Ellermann JM, Ludwig KD, Nissi MJ, Johnson CP, Strupp JP, Wang L, et al. Three-dimensional quantitative magnetic resonance imaging of epiphyseal cartilage vascularity using vessel image features: New insights into juvenile osteochondritis dissecans. JBJS Open Access. 2019;**4**(4):e0031.1-9

[26] Wilson JN. A diagnostic sign in osteochondritis dissecans of the knee. Journal of Bone Joint Surgery American. 1967;**49**(3):477-480

[27] Cruz AI, Shea KG, Ganley TJ. Pediatric Knee Osteochondritis Dissecans Lesions. Orthopedic Clinics of North America. 2016;**47**(4):763-775

[28] de Smet AA, Fisher DR, Graf BK, Lange RH. Osteochondritis dissecans of the knee: Value of MR imaging in determining lesion stability and the presence of articular cartilage defects. American Journal of Roentgenology. 1990;**155**(3):549-553

[29] Kijowski R, Blankenbaker DG, Shinki K, Fine JP, Graf BK, de Smet AA. Juvenile versus adult osteochondritis

dissecans of the knee: Appropriate MR imaging criteria for instability. Radiology. 2008;**248**(2):571-578

[30] Moktassi A, Popkin CA, White LM, Murnaghan ML. Imaging of osteochondritis dissecans. Orthopedic Clinical North America. 2012;**43**(2):201-211

[31] Ruchelsman DE, Hall MR, Youm T. Osteochondritis dissecans of the capitellum: Current concepts. Journal of American Academy Orthopedic Surgery. 2010;**18**(9):557-567

[32] Li X, Johnson CP, Ellermann J. Measuring Knee Bone Marrow Perfusion Using Arterial Spin Labeling at 3 T. Scientific Reports. 2020;**10**:5260. DOI: 10.1038/s41598-020-62110-y

[33] de Smet AA, Ilahi OA, Graf BK. Reassessment of the MR criteria for stability of osteochondritis dissecans in the knee and ankle. Skeletal Radiology. 1996;**25**(2):159-163

[34] Brittberg M, Winalski CS. Evaluation of cartilage injuries and repair. Journal of Bone Joint Surgery American. 2003;**2**:58-69

[35] Guhl JF. Arthroscopic treatment of osteochondritis dissecans: Preliminary report. The Orthopedic Clinics of North America. 1979;**10**(3):671-683

[36] Dipaola JD, Nelson DW, Colville MR. Characterizing osteochondral lesions by magnetic resonance imaging. Arthroscopy: The Journal of Arthroscopic and Related Surgery. 1991;**7**(1):101-104

[37] Wall EJ, Vourazeris J, Myer GD, Emery KH, Divine JG, Nick TG, et al. The healing potential of stable juvenile osteochondritis dissecans knee lesions. Journal of Bone and Joint Surgery - Series A. 2008;**90**(12):2655-2664

[38] Krause M, Hapfelmeier A, Möller M, Amling M, Bohndorf K, Meenen NM. Healing predictors of stable juvenile osteochondritis dissecans knee lesions after 6 and 12 months of nonoperative treatment. The American Journal of Sports Medicine. 2013;**41**(10):2384-2391

[39] Hughes JA, Cook J. Juvenile osteochondritis dissecans: A 5-year review of the natural history using clinical and MRI evaluation. Pediatric Radiology. 2003;**33**(6):410-417

[40] Jürgensen I, Bachmann G, Schleicher I, Haas H. Arthroscopic Versus Conservative Treatment of Osteochondritis. Arthroscopy. 2002;**18**(4):378-386

[41] Cahill BR, Ahten SM. The three critical components in the conservative treatment of juvenile osteochondritis dissecans (JOCD): Physician, parent, and child. Clinics in Sports Medicine. 2001;**20**(2):287-298

[42] Sanders TL, Pareek A, Johnson NR, Carey JL, Maak TG, Stuart MJ, et al. Nonoperative management of osteochondritis dissecans of the knee: Progression to osteoarthritis and arthroplasty at mean 13-year follow-up. Orthop. The Journal of Sports Medicine. 2017;**5**(7):2325967117704644

[43] Sanders TL, Pareek A, Obey MR, Johnson NR, Carey JL, Stuart MJ, et al. High rate of osteoarthritis after osteochondritis dissecans fragment excision compared with surgical restoration at a mean 16-Year Follow-up. The American Journal of Sports Medicine. 2017;**45**(8):1799-1805

[44] Ytrehus B, Carlson CS, Ekman S. Etiology and pathogenesis of

osteochondrosis. Veterinary Pathology. 2007;**44**(4):429-448

[45] Gunton MJ, Carey JL, Shaw CR, Murnaghan ML. Drilling juvenile osteochondritis dissecans: Retro- or transarticular? Knee: Clinical Orthopedic Related Research. 2013;**471**(4):1144-1151

[46] Louisia S, Beaufils P, Katabi M, Robert H. Transchondral drilling for osteochondritis dissecans of the medial condyle of the knee. Knee Surgery, Sports Traumatology, Arthroscopy. 2003;**11**(1):33-39

[47] Semenov A et al. Surgical treatment of stable foci of the osteochondritis dissecans in children: A systematic review. Detskaya Khirurgiya. 2021;**25**(3):179

[48] Leland DP, Bernard CD, Camp CL. Does Internal Fixation for Unstable Osteochondritis Systematic Review. Arthroscopy: The Journal of Arthroscopic and Related Surgery. 2019;**35**(8):2512-2522

[49] Kocher MS, Czarnecki JJ, Andersen JS, Micheli LJ. Internal fixation of juvenile osteochondritis dissecans lesions of the knee. The American Journal of Sports Medicine. 2007;**35**(5):712-718

[50] Ishikawa M, Nakamae A, Nakasa T, Ikuta Y, Hayashi S, Ochi M, et al. Limitation of in-situ arthroscopic fixation for stable juvenile osteochondritis dissecans in the knee. Journal of Pediatric Orthopaedics Part B. 2018;**27**(6):516-521

[51] Wu IT, Custers RJH, Desai VS, Pareek A, Stuart MJ, Saris DBF, et al. Internal fixation of unstable Osteochondritis Dissecans: Do open growth plates improve healing rate? The American Journal of Sports Medicine. 2018;**46**(10):2394-2401

[52] Hinckel BB, Thomas D, Vellios EE, Hancock KJ, Calcei JG, Sherman SL, et al. Algorithm for treatment of focal cartilage defects of the knee: Classic and new procedures. Cartilage. 2021;**13**(1):473S-495S

[53] Bekkers JEJ, Inklaar M, Saris DBF. Treatment selection in articular cartilage lesions of the knee: A systematic review. American Journal of Sports Medicine. 2009;**37**:148S-155S

[54] Solheim E, Hegna J, Inderhaug E, Øyen J, Harlem T, Strand T. Results at 10-14 years after microfracture treatment of articular cartilage defects in the knee. Knee Surgery, Sports Traumatology, Arthroscopy. 2016;**24**(5):1587-1593

[55] Frisbie DD, Oxford JT, Southwood L, Trotter GW, Rodkey WG, Steadman JR, et al. Early events in cartilage repair after subchondral bone microfracture. Clinical Orthopedic Related Research. 2003;**407**:215-227

[56] Minas T, Nehrer S. Current concepts in the treatment of articular cartilage defects. Orthopedics. 1997;**20**(6):525-538

[57] Kraeutler MJ, Aliberti GM, Scillia AJ, McCarty EC, Mulcahey MK. Microfracture versus drilling of articular cartilage defects: A systematic review of the basic science evidence. Orthopaedic Journal of Sports Medicine. 2020;**8**(8):1-7

[58] Chen H, Hoemann CD, Sun J, Chevrier A, McKee MD, Shive MS, et al. Depth of subchondral perforation influences the outcome of bone marrow stimulation cartilage repair. Journal of Orthopaedic Research. 2011;**29**(8):1178-1184

[59] Chen H, Chevrier A, Hoemann CD, Sun J, Ouyang W, Buschmann MD. Characterization of subchondral bone repair for marrow-stimulated

chondral defects and its relationship to articular cartilage resurfacing. The American Journal of Sports Medicine. 2011;**39**(8):1731-1740

[60] Pareek A, Reardon PJ, Macalena JA, Levy BA, Stuart MJ, Williams RJ, et al. Osteochondral Autograft transfer versus microfracture in the knee: A meta-analysis of prospective comparative studies at midterm. Arthroscopy: The Journal of Arthroscopic and Related Surgery. 2016;**32**(10):2118-2130

[61] Krych AJ, Harnly HW, Rodeo SA, Williams RJ. Activity levels are higher after osteochondral autograft transfer mosaicplasty than after microfracture for articular cartilage defects of the knee: A retrospective comparative study. Journal of Bone Joint Surgical American. 2012;**94**(11):971-978

[62] GudasR,SimonaityteR,ČekanauskasE, Tamošiunas R. A prospective, randomized clinical study of osteochondral autologous transplantation versus microfracture for the treatment of osteochondritis dissecans in the knee joint in children. Journal of Pediatric Orthopaedics. 2009;**29**(7):741-748

[63] Solheim E, Hegna J, Strand T, Harlem T, Inderhaug E. Randomized study of Long-term (15-17 Years) outcome after microfracture versus mosaicplasty in knee articular cartilage defects. The American Journal of Sports Medicine. 2018;**46**(4):826-831

[64] Pareek A, Reardon PJ, Maak TG, Levy BA, Stuart MJ, Krych AJ. Long-term outcomes after osteochondral autograft transfer: A systematic review at mean follow-up of 10.2 years. Arthroscopy - Journal of Arthroscopic and Related Surgery. 2016;**32**:1174-1184

[65] Basad E, Ishaque B, Bachmann G, Stürz H, Steinmeyer J. Matrix-induced autologous chondrocyte implantation versus microfracture in the treatment of cartilage defects of the knee: A 2-year randomised study. Knee Surgery, Sports Traumatology, Arthroscopy. 2010;**18**(4):519-527

[66] Brittberg M, Recker D, Ilgenfritz J, Saris DBF. Matrix-applied characterized autologous cultured chondrocytes versus microfracture: Five-year follow-up of a prospective randomized trial. The American Journal of Sports Medicine. 2018;**46**(6):1343-1351

[67] Volz M, Schaumburger J, Frick H, Grifka J, Anders S. A randomized controlled trial demonstrating sustained benefit of Autologous Matrix-Induced Chondrogenesis over microfracture at five years. International Orthopaedics. 2017;**41**(4):797-804

[68] de Girolamo L, Schönhuber H, Viganò M, Bait C, Quaglia A, Thiebat G, et al. Autologous Matrix-Induced Chondrogenesis (AMIC) and AMIC enhanced by autologous concentrated Bone Marrow Aspirate (BMAC) Allow for stable clinical and functional improvements at up to 9 years follow-up: Results from a Randomized controlled study. Journal of Clinical Medicine. 2019;**8**(3):392

[69] Gille J, Schuseil E, Wimmer J, Gellissen J, Schulz AP, Behrens P. Mid-term results of autologous matrix induced chondrogenesis for treatment of focal cartilage defects in the knee. Knee Surgery, Sports Traumatology, Arthroscopy. 2010;**18**(11):1456-1464

[70] Salzmann GM, Ossendorff R, Gilat R, Cole BJ. Autologous minced cartilage implantation for treatment of chondral and osteochondral lesions in the knee joint: An overview. Cartilage. 2021;**13**:1124S-1136S

[71] Levinson C, Cavalli E, Sindi DM, Kessel B, Zenobi-Wong M, Preiss S, et al. Chondrocytes from device-minced articular cartilage show potent outgrowth into fibrin and collagen hydrogels. The Journal of Sports Medicine. 2019;**7**(9):2325967119867618

[72] Salzmann GM, Niemeyer P, Hochrein A, Stoddart MJ, Angele P. Articular cartilage repair of the knee in children and adolescents. The Journal of Sports Medicine. 2018;**6**(3):2325967118760190

[73] Bonasia DE, Marmotti A, Mattia S, Cosentino A, Spolaore S, Governale G, et al. The degree of chondral fragmentation affects extracellular matrix production in cartilage autograft implantation: An in vitro study. Arthroscopy: The Journal of Arthroscopic and Related Surgery. 2015;**31**(12):2335-2341

[74] Runer A, Salzmann GM. Moving towards single stage cartilage repair—is there evidence for the minced cartilage procedure? Journal of Cartilage & Joint Preservation. 2022;**2**(2):100053

[75] Lu Y, Dhanaraj S, Wang Z, Bradley DM, Bowman SM, Cole BJ, et al. Minced cartilage without cell culture serves as an effective intraoperative cell source for cartilage repair. Journal of Orthopaedic Research. 2006;**24**(6):1261-1270

[76] Cole BJ, Farr J, Winalski CS, Hosea T, Richmond J, Mandelbaum B, et al. Outcomes after a single-stage procedure for cell-based cartilage repair: A prospective clinical safety trial with 2-year follow-up. The American Journal of Sports Medicine. 2011;**39**(6):1170-1179

[77] Schneider S, Ossendorff R, Holz J, Salzmann GM. Arthroscopic Minced Cartilage Implantation (MCI): A Technical Note. Arthroscopy Techniques. 2021;**10**(1):e97-e101

[78] Christensen BB, Foldager CB, Jensen J, Lind M. Autologous dual-tissue transplantation for osteochondral repair: Early clinical and radiological results. Cartilage. 2015;**6**(3):166-173

[79] Massen FK, Inauen CR, Harder LP, Runer A, Preiss S, Salzmann GM. One-step autologous minced cartilage procedure for the treatment of knee joint chondral and osteochondral lesions: A series of 27 patients with 2-year follow-up. Orthopedic Journal of Sports Medicine. 2019;**7**(6):2325967119853773

[80] Cugat R, Alentorn-Geli E, Navarro J, Cuscó X, Steinbacher G, Seijas R, et al. A novel autologous-made matrix using hyaline cartilage chips and platelet-rich growth factors for the treatment of full-thickness cartilage or osteochondral defects: Preliminary results. Journal of Orthopedic Surgery. 2020;**28**(1):2309499019887547

[81] Bonasia DE, Martin JA, Marmotti A, Amendola RL, Buckwalter JA, Rossi R, et al. Cocultures of adult and juvenile chondrocytes compared with adult and juvenile chondral fragments: In vitro matrix production. American Journal of Sports Medicine. 2011;**39**(11):2355-2361

[82] Adkisson HD, Martin JA, Amendola RL, Milliman C, Mauch KA, Katwal AB, et al. The potential of human allogeneic juvenile chondrocytes for restoration of articular cartilage. American Journal of Sports Medicine. 2010;**38**(7):1324-1333

[83] Ao Y, Li Z, You Q, Zhang C, Yang L, Duan X. The use of particulated juvenile allograft cartilage for the repair of porcine articular cartilage defects. American Journal of Sports Medicine. 2019;**47**(10):2308-2315

[84] Gruber R, Varga F, Fischer MB, Watzek G. Platelets

stimulate proliferation of bone cells: Involvement of platelet-derived growth factor, microparticles and membranes. Clinical Oral Implants Research. 2002;**13**(5):529-535

[85] Delong JM, Russell RP, Mazzocca AD. Platelet-rich plasma: The PAW classification system. Arthroscopy. 2012;**28**(7):998-1009

[86] Shahid M, Kundra R. Platelet-rich plasma (PRP) for knee disorders. EFORT Open Review. 2017;**2**:28-34

[87] Dragoo JL, Guzman RA. Evaluation of the consistency and composition of commercially available bone marrow aspirate concentrate systems. The Journal of Sports Medicine. 2020;**8**(1):2325967119893634

[88] Sharma DK, Kumar N. Osteochondritis dissecans—Does platelet rich plasma really help. Journal of Clinical Orthopedic Trauma. 2018;**9**(2):153-156

[89] Davidson K, Grimm NL, Christino MA, Willimon SC, Busch MT. Retroarticular drilling with supplemental bone marrow aspirate concentrate for the treatment of osteochondritis dissecans of the knee. The Journal of Sports Medicine. 2018;**4**(7):232

[90] Andelman SM, Mandelbaum BR, Fitzsimmons KP, Pace JL. Retroarticular core decompression with biologic augmentation for juvenile osteochondritis dissecans of the knee. Arthroscopy Technical. 2020;**9**(7):e1003-e1009

[91] Baldassarri M, Buda R, Perazzo L, Ghinelli D, Sarino R, Grigolo B, et al. Osteocondritis dissecans lesions of the knee restored by bone marrow aspirate concentrate. Clinical and imaging results in 18 patients. European Journal of Orthopaedic Surgery and Traumatology. 8 Feb 2022. DOI: 10.1007/s00590-022-03214-1. Epub ahead of print. PMID: 35133501

[92] Bausset O, Giraudo L, Veran J, Magalon J, Coudreuse JM, Magalon G, et al. Formulation and storage of platelet-rich plasma homemade product. Bioresearch Open Access. 2012;**1**(3):115-123

[93] Wall EJ, Milewski MD, Carey JL, Shea KG, Ganley TJ, Polousky JD, et al. The reliability of assessing radiographic healing of osteochondritis dissecans of the knee. The American Journal of Sports Medicine. 2017;**45**(6):1370-1375

[94] Parikh SN, Allen M, Wall EJ, May MM, Laor T, Zbojniewicz AM, et al. The reliability to determine 'healing' in osteochondritis dissecans from radiographic assessment. Journal of Pediatric Orthopaedics. 2012;**32**(6):35-39

[95] Semenov A et al. Reliability of the novel MRI-based OCD lesion healing assessment tool for adolescent OCD of the knee. Pediatric Traumatology, Orthopaedics and Reconstructive Surgery. 2022;**10**(1):57-70

[96] Hevesi M, Sanders TL, Pareek A, Milbrandt TA, Levy BA, Stuart MJ, et al. Osteochondritis dissecans in the knee of skeletally immature patients: Rates of persistent pain, osteoarthritis, and arthroplasty at mean 14-years' follow-up. Cartilage. 2018

[97] Abouassaly M, Peterson D, Salci L, Farrokhyar F, D'Souza J, Bhandari M, et al. Surgical management of osteochondritis dissecans of the knee in the paediatric population: A systematic review addressing surgical techniques. Knee Surgery, Sports Traumatology, Arthroscopy. 2014;**22**(6):1216-1224

[98] Edmonds EW, Albright J, Bastrom T, Chambers HG. Outcomes of extra-articular, intra-epiphyseal drilling for osteochondritis dissecans of the knee. Journal of Pediatric Orthopaedics. 2010;**30**(8):870-878

[99] Lee CS, Larsen CG, Marchwiany DA, Chudik SC. Extra-articular, intraepiphyseal drilling for osteochondritis dissecans of the knee: Characterization of a safe and reproducible surgical approach. The Journal of Sports Medicine. 2019;7(2):2325967119830397

[100] Anderson AF, Richards DB, Pagnani MJ, Hovis WD. Antegrade drilling for osteochondritis dissecans of the knee. Arthroscopy. 1997;**13**(3):319-324

[101] Hayan R, Phillipe G, Ludovic S, Claude K, Jean-Michel C. Juvenile osteochondritis of femoral condyles: Treatment with transchondral drilling. Analysis of 40 cases. Journal of Children's Orthopaedics. 2010;**4**(1):39-44

[102] Marmotti A, Rossi R, Castoldi F, Roveda E, Michielon G, Peretti GM. PRP and articular cartilage: A clinical update. BioMed Research International. 2015;**2015**:542502

[103] Kobayashi E, Flückiger L, Fujioka-Kobayashi M, Sawada K, Sculean A, Schaller B, et al. Comparative release of growth factors from PRP, PRF, and advanced-PRF. Clinical Oral Investigations. 2016;**20**(9):2353-2360

[104] Dohan Ehrenfest DM, Andia I, Zumstein MA, Zhang CQ, Pinto NR, Bielecki T. Classification of platelet concentrates (Platelet-Rich Plasma-PRP, platelet-rich fibrin-PRF) for topical and infiltrative use in orthopedic and sports medicine: Current consensus, clinical implications and perspectives. Muscles, Ligaments and Tendons Journal. 2014;**4**:3-9

[105] Bielecki T, Gazdzik TS, Szczepanski T. Benefit of percutaneous injection of autologous platelet-leukocyte-rich gel in patients with delayed union and nonunion. European Surgical Research. 2008;**40**(3):289-296

[106] Redondo ML, Beer AJ, Yanke AB. Cartilage restoration: Microfracture and osteochondral autograft transplantation. The Journal of Knee Surgery. 2018;**31**(3):231-238

[107] Versier G, Dubrana F. Treatment of knee cartilage defect in 2010. Orthopaedics & Traumatology, Surgery & Research. 2011;**97**(8 SUPPL):140-153

[108] Numata H, Nakase J, Oshima T, Tsuchiya H. Effectiveness of adhering adipose-derived stem cells to defective cartilage in promoting cartilage regeneration in a rabbit model. Arthroscopy - Journal of Arthroscopic and Related Surgery. 2019;**53**:1-8

[109] Jungmann PM, Gersing AS, Baumann F, Holwein C, Braun S, Neumann J, et al. Cartilage repair surgery prevents progression of knee degeneration. Knee Surgery, Sports Traumatology, Arthroscopy. 2019;(9):3001-3013

[110] Yoon TH, Jung M, Choi CH, Kim HS, Lee YH, Choi YS, et al. Arthroscopic gel-type autologous chondrocyte implantation presents histologic evidence of regenerating hyaline-like cartilage in the knee with articular cartilage defect. Knee Surgery, Sports Traumatology, Arthroscopy. 2020;(3):941-951

[111] Cotter EJ, Wang KC, Yanke AB, Chubinskaya S. Bone marrow aspirate concentrate for cartilage defects of the knee: From Bench to Bedside Evidence. Cartilage. 2018;**9**:161-170

[112] Tsuyuguchi Y, Nakasa T, Ishikawa M, Miyaki S, Matsushita R,

Kanemitsu M, et al. The benefit of minced cartilage over isolated chondrocytes in atelocollagen gel on chondrocyte proliferation and migration. Cartilage. 2021;**12**(1):93-101

[113] Karpinski K, Häner M, Bierke S, Petersen W. Matrix-induced chondrogenesis is a valid and safe cartilage repair option for small- to medium-sized cartilage defects of the knee: A systematic review. Knee Surgery, Sports Traumatology, Arthroscopy. 2021;**29**:4213-4222

Chapter 6

Distal Femoral Fractures

Renzo Reyes, María González-Alonso, Samer Amhaz-Escanlar, Alberto De Castro, Jesús Pino-Mínguez and Alberto Jorge-Mora

Abstract

Distal femur fractures are increasing injuries in our environment, due to their close relationship with the aging of the population. The diagnosis and treatment of these injuries have evolved in recent years, and the availability of new tools allows us to improve the results of our patients. Techniques such as dual nail-plate or plate-plate fixation emerge as an option in complications and complex fractures, and augmentation with PMMA may be an option in very low-density bones. To use these new techniques, anatomical knowledge, especially of the medial aspect of the femur, is essential. Many recent publications have studied the use of minimally invasive techniques with safe pathways. Throughout the following pages, we give a glimpse of the novelties in the treatment of these fractures, and we review the classic concepts.

Keywords: distal femur, fracture, fixation, PMMA, nailing, plating

1. Introduction

Although distal femur fractures represent <1% of all fractures, an increase in their incidence has been observed in relation to the aging of the population [1–3]. Studies completed in developed countries show a general incidence rate of distal femur fractures that ranges between 4.7 and 8.7 fractures per 100,000 patients per year [1–3].

These types of fractures have a bimodal distribution. There is a peak in young adults, often men, which decreases until the age of 50 in relation to high-energy polytrauma. This peak has been progressively decreasing in direct relation to the development of safety mechanisms in vehicles and currently represents a low fraction of all fractures [2]. As a result of high-energy injury mechanisms, percentages of open fractures close to 20% have been reported, especially in relation to traffic accidents and occupational accidents, and the presence of a high-energy distal femoral fracture should aware us of associated injuries [4]. A common mechanism in traffic accidents associated with this group of age is the "dashboard injury" in which the patella strikes the knee like a wedge between the femoral condyles. This pattern is associated with a higher risk of additional fractures in the ipsilateral extremity, particularly in patella, tibia and fibula, hip, and acetabulum, as well as non-orthopaedic injuries as damage in trunk and skull [4].

These fractures have a high mortality rate in the set of a high-energy trauma at 30 days, 6 months, and 1 year which are 1%, 2%, and 3%, respectively [5].

From the age of 60, we found an increase in mortality for both sexes with a female predominance in relation to low-energy trauma that could be comparable to hip or femoral shaft fractures in the elderly. The overall incidence rate in people over 60 years of age is 43 per 100,000 patients per year in men and 217 in women [5]. In this population group, the mortality rate at 30 days, 6 months and 1 year amounts to 8%, 26%, and 35%, respectively, and this increase is related to the age of the patient and their comorbidities [5].

Due to the high number of knee replacements performed, another type of distal femur fractures consisting of periprosthetic fractures is standing out. Due to their biological and mechanical characteristics, they constitute a clearly differentiated subgroup. The frequency of periprosthetic fractures of the distal femur after total knee arthroplasty is reported to be between 0.3 and 5.5% for primary knee arthroplasties and up to 30% after a revision procedure [6, 7]. In these patients, the annual mortality rate is 15% [5].

Extra-articular supracondylar fractures are the most frequent fractures, followed by partial articular fractures and complex supra-intercondylar fractures [3].

2. Anatomy

There have been proposed different descriptions to define the limits that involve the distal femur, but one of the most used is to define the distal femur as a square segment with a side distance equivalent to the space between both epicondiles (**Figure 1**).

This segment is particularly relevant for several reasons as follows:

- It is part of the knee joint, and injuries to it will affect its mechanics and kinematics.
- Together with the proximal tibia, it constitutes the segment of the lower extremity that is most affected by malunion, so a nonanatomical reduction will modify the axes of the extremity in a higher degree.

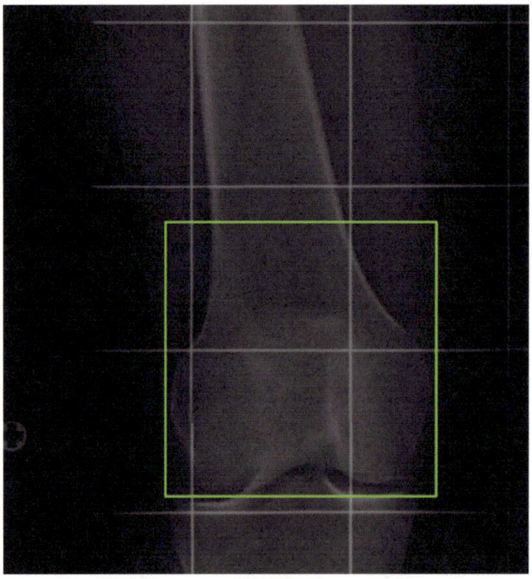

Figure 1.
Segment that defines the distal femur.

- It is a joint whose stability and congruence depend on several elements, highlighting the ligamentous complexes, the menisci and the extensor apparatus of the knee. The repair and preservation of these structures are essential to preserve the function of the knee, and many injuries to the distal femur will compromise them.

If we focus on the shape, we see that the diaphysis of the distal femur widens into a cone shape with a trapezoidal projection corresponding to the medial and lateral condyles [8, 9]. The medial femoral condyle is larger and extends distally compared to the lateral femoral condyle [10]. For this reason, the anatomical axis of the distal femur, which is formed between the distal joint line and the diaphyseal axis, has 6–11° of valgus (**Figure 2**) [10, 11]. The lateral and medial cortex are inclined about 25° and 10°, respectively, in the axial plane toward the midline, which will condition the insertion of osteosynthesis material in this area. The posterior halves of the condyles are posterior to the posterior cortex of the femur [12].

Between both condyles is the intercondylar fossa. Each of the faces contributed by the condyles to this groove constitutes the insertion of the cruciate ligaments, the one offered by the lateral condyle for the anterior and the medial one for the posterior. The point anterior to the proximal insertion of the anterior cruciate ligament corresponds to the distal point of Blumensaat's line and is the entry portal for the retrograde intramedullary nail (**Figure 3**).

The medial and lateral collateral ligaments emerge from the medial and lateral epicondyles, respectively.

Surrounding the femur, we find a large part of the muscles that contribute to the mobility of the lower extremity, causing in cases of fracture the displacement of the bone fragments and conditioning deformity depending on the place of the fracture (**Figure 4**):

- Quadriceps and hamstrings favor shortening.

- The adductors help shortening and can promote varus disaxation, especially if there is metaphyseal comminution.

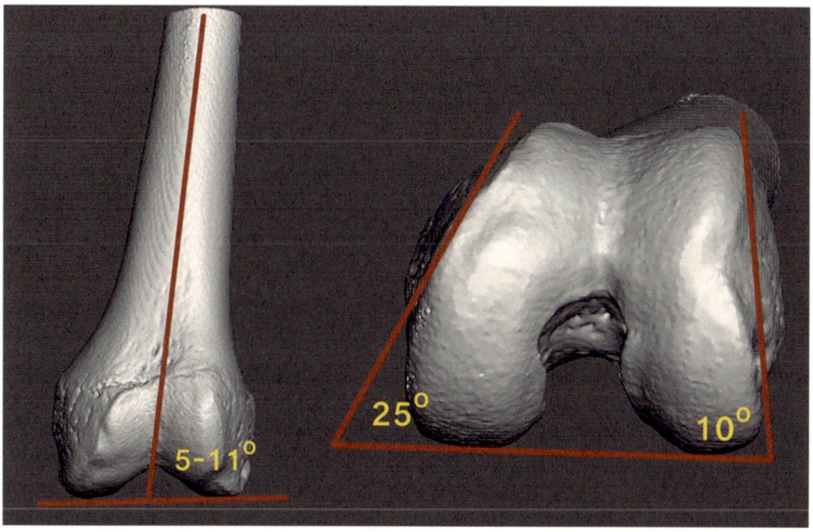

Figure 2.
Angles of the distal femur.

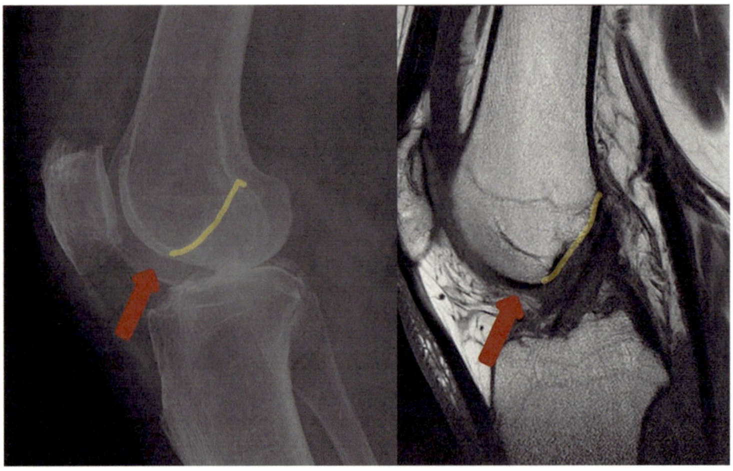

Figure 3.
Entry point for distal femoral nailing and its relation to the anterior cruciate ligament. In yellow the Blumensaat's line.

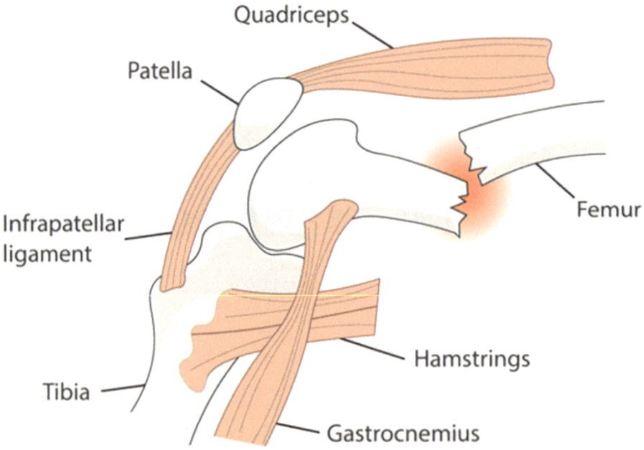

Figure 4.
Deformity forces in distal femoral fractures.

- The gastrocnemius causes a deformity with posterior apex of the distal fragment that can compromise the neurovascular bundle 11.

The position of the vascular bundle in the distal femur favored ruling out approaches other than the anterior and lateral ones (**Figure 5**). Recently, thanks to the evolution in surgical knowledge of the area, the development of anatomical materials, and the need to improve fixation in these complex fractures, medial approaches to the distal femur with proximal extension have been developed. To be able to carry them out, abundant studies have been completed on cadavers for percutaneous techniques and with a special interest in the Hunter's canal. Interesting is the study by Maslow that focuses on seeing how far the femoral artery passes from the anterior to the posterior area of the femur, describing a mean distance from the adductor tubercle to the femoral artery of 23.2 cm and 14.3 cm at the level of the anterior border and posterior femur, respectively. This would allow us to use percutaneous plates using this safety distance. In open surgery, the location of the geniculate artery allows us to control it

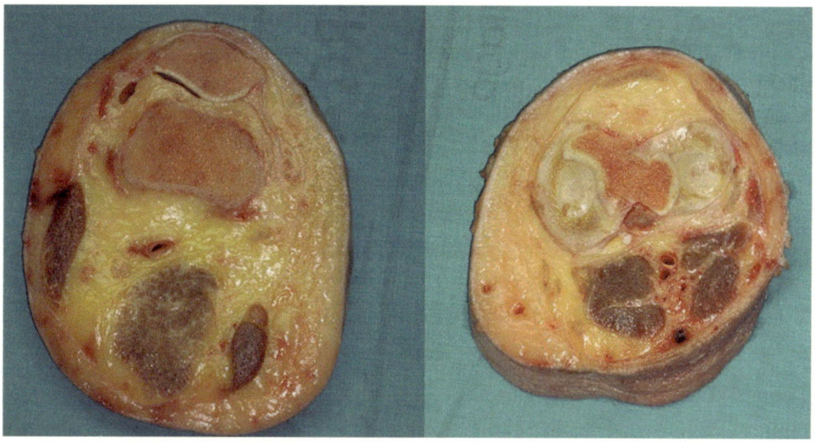

Figure 5.
Distal femoral anatomy in sagittal anatomical images.

to unhook the package and favor access. The descending geniculate artery originates at a mean of 10.8 cm from the adductor tubercle [13]. It should always be kept in mind that the intraoperative position may vary in relation to the trauma.

Knowledge of this vascular anatomy will also allow us to play with the implantation of cerclages in safe areas or choose the best approaches to access risk areas.

3. Diagnosis

The diagnosis of a distal femur fracture is usually clear in most cases, finding young patients with high-energy trauma with obvious deformity or older patients with less deformity, but with pain and ecchymosis that facilitate the diagnosis, which

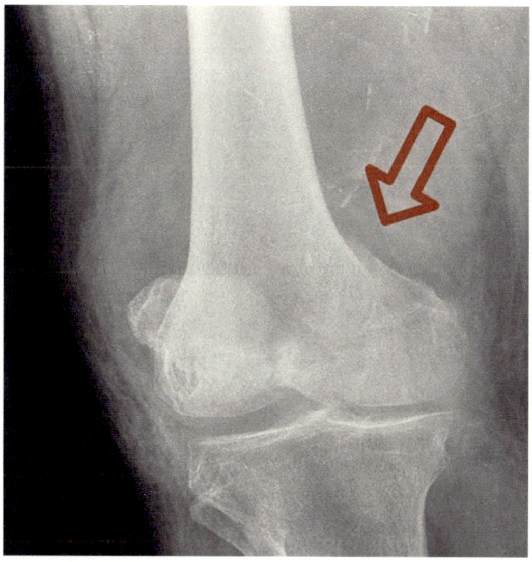

Figure 6.
Coronal shear fracture is seen on an oblique view.

is easily confirmed on a two-plane radiological test. Basic radiological studies should include simple radiographs of the total femur to rule out the presence of acetabular, hip, femoral diaphyseal, patella, and hip dislocation or fractures. If there is excessive shortening or deformity, traction views can help the study [14]. In those situations, with partial fractures, especially in the coronal planes, the diagnosis is complicated. In these cases, functional limitation and hemarthrosis should lead us to a joint injury that will force us to perform oblique radiographs to confirm the injury (**Figure 6**). In many cases, performing a CT will allow us to complete the diagnosis and will provide us with information on the complex three-dimensional structure of the distal femur, especially in trauma with joint comminution.

The use of MRI is generally restricted when chondral, tendon, meniscal, and ligamentous injuries associated with trauma are suspected. It is especially useful in knee instabilities and injuries of the extensor apparatus since they frequently accompany high-energy trauma.

We must also know the vascular status of the limb and suspect an injury in the presence of any of the four signs of vascular injuries, such as pulsatile hemorrhage, expanding hematoma, palpable thrill/audible murmur, or a pulseless limb. When these four signs are present, immediate surgical exploration is warranted. In patients with one of the four signs, an ankle-brachial index is recommended. If this is greater than 0.9, a clinical follow-up can be carried out without further studies. If it is less than or equal to 0.9, arteriography or Doppler ultrasound should be performed [15].

4. Fracture classification

Currently, the AO/OTA classification (**Figure 7**) is the most widely used classification in clinical practice and research, since it allows the use of an alphanumeric coding system

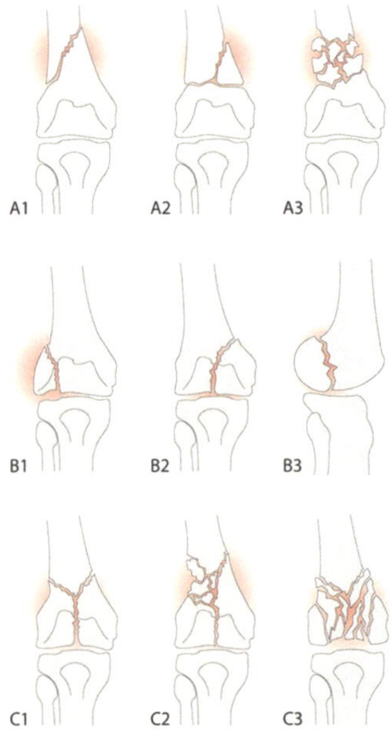

Figure 7.
AO classification.

that facilitates data storage and provides a hierarchy of severity [16]. Code 33 is designated for the location of this fracture. In addition, these fractures are divided into extra-articular (type A), partial articular or unicondylar (type B), and intra-articular (type C) [10]. Subgroups from 1 to 3 provide information on the degree of comminution in types A and C fractures. In type B fractures, however, the subgroups refer to the pattern of the fracture; type B1 are sagittal fractures of the lateral condyle, type B2 are sagittal fractures of the medial condyle, and type B3 are coronal fractures known as Hoffa's fractures, described in 1907 and usually affect the lateral condyle [17].

5. Management

The results published in recent years lead us to consider that distal femur fractures are always surgical, except in limited cases, due to the high mortality associated with conservative management and the number of complications, such as knee stiffness, inadequate alignment, consolidation delays, soft tissue problems, and prolonged hospitalization [18, 19].

There are few exceptions to this rule, more related to the patient than to the fracture itself. In recent years, the following situations have been described that may be considered relative contraindications, since even in these cases surgery may be beneficial: very high-surgical risk that prevents anesthesia, non-displaced fractures, non-ambulant patients, and irreversible spinal cord injuries [10, 20].

The fundamental objectives of surgery will be to achieve a good reduction of the joint surfaces, maintain the length of the femur, as well as alignment and rotation; achieving knee stability that allows rapid mobilization [9]. Stabilization in the sagittal plane with rotation of the condyles, unlike stabilization in the frontal plane, represents a challenge for the surgeon [21].

In high-energy fractures with comminution and shortening, unstable fractures, open fractures, fractures with vascular injury, or in the context of damage control orthopedics in polytraumatized patients, the use of a temporary external fixator will be useful until surgery is performed. Trans-skeletal traction can be useful for short waiting periods, but it is in disuse due to the limitation it entails for the management and care of hospitalized patients.

6. Fracture fixation and approaches

In most distal femur fractures, we will opt for a radiolucent table position, with supports and pads that allow correcting the deformity of the fracture (**Figure 8**). We must count on the elevation of the knee to angle the beam of rays and achieve correct orthogonal projections. It is also essential to allow access to the contralateral limb and hips, to compare length and rotation between limbs. To control screw lengthening, we should consider distal femoral angulations shown in **Figure 2** to angulate the x-ray beam to fit both angles.

Another point of concern is rotation adjustment. In complex, distal femoral fractures are challenging. We have several tools to confirm this rotation: use of lesser trochanter, clinical rotation, and femoral cortex reduction, but the use of the lesser trochanter profile seems to be useful and reliable [22].

There are different approaches that will allow us to treat injuries of the distal femur.

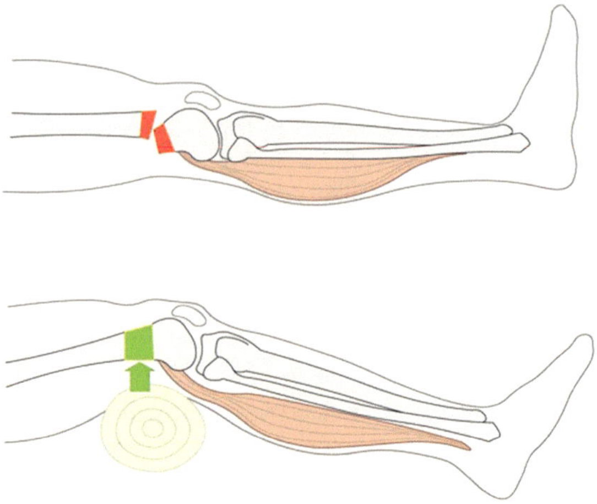

Figure 8.
Reduction of deformity in distal femoral fractures.

In extra-articular or simple partial articular fractures, we can choose minimally invasive techniques, through lateral approaches or nailing techniques.

In case of complex joint injuries, joint exposure is necessary. In these cases, we can opt for parapatellar approaches, among which the external one is the most used, or techniques such as the TARPO approach, Swashbuckler, Olerud extensible anterior, and window approaches that allow us greater control of the joint fragments. If we need to provide medial support to prevent varus collapse, medial approaches will be necessary. On many occasions, especially in open fractures, we must adapt our approach to the underlying situation and minimize the damage to healthy structures by repairing the damaged ones (**Figure 9**).

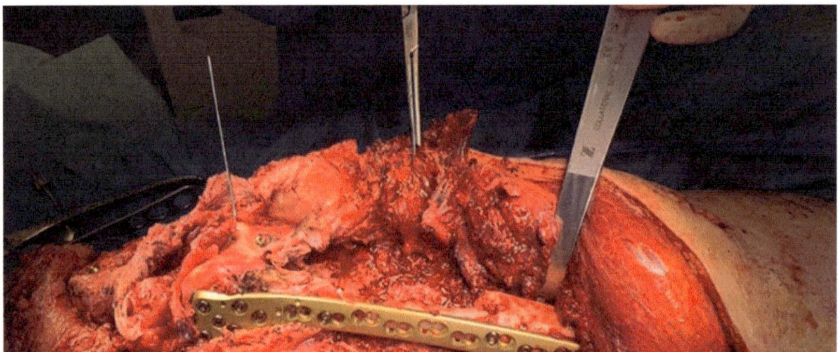

Figure 9.
Extensile modified lateral approach in a patient with a bone defect and a complete injury of the extensor mechanism.

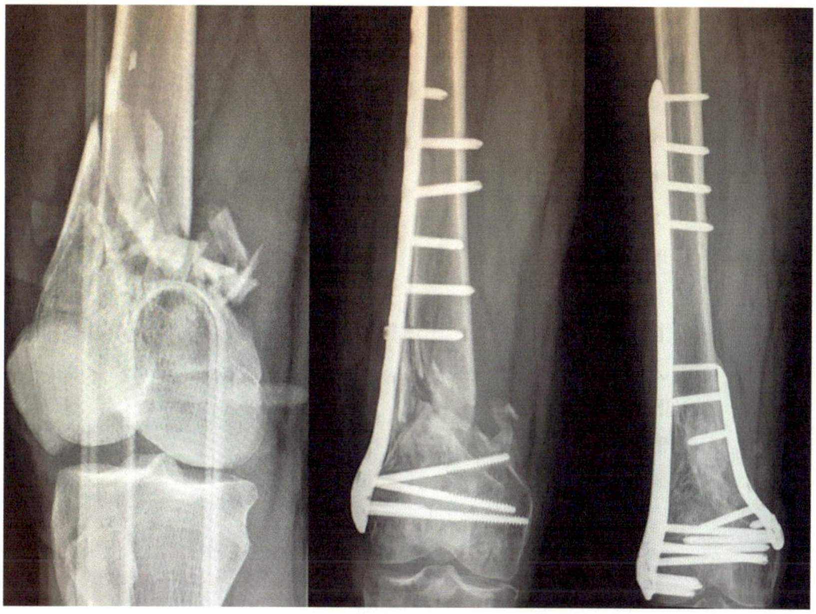

Figure 10.
Distal comminuted fracture treated with a lateral plate. Failed fixation was rescued with a double plate fixation.

To achieve a proper fracture fixation, we must always follow certain principles that allow us to achieve good results in any situation. For this reason, we must follow a strategy that must consist of gradually reducing the complexity of the injury: we will begin by reconstructing the joint block, to later neutralize and fix the metaphyseal area.

The distal femur is going to be subjected to torsional forces and a lot of axial load, which will condition a high varus stress [21]. If we anticipate long consolidation times, sometimes a lateral plate does not tolerate the situation and suffers from fatigue, and the use of medial plates or intramedullary nails with or without a lateral plate will provide additional fixation that will improve our results (**Figure 10**) [23].

We are going to face special situations, in which the complexity of the injury is going to force us to increase our fixation to prevent early collapse. Perhaps the osteoporotic fracture is today our battle horse, with fragile bones that prevent the adequate purchase and load transmission to the implant, leading to early failure and limiting the mobility of patients who require early loading. In these cases, the use of PMMA (**Figure 11**) to improve the bone-screw interface will give us a plus that can solve extreme cases [24].

In the case of type B fractures (partial joints), total stability is required, for which interfragmentary compression would be necessary, normally with compression screws; to which another buttress plate can be added (**Figure 12**) [14]. As specific indications for the use of locked plates, we find comminution and poor bone stock [25].

Distal femoral replacement involves resection of the supracondylar segment of the femur and replacement with a rotational hinge knee system [26]. The main objective of the treatment when treating distal femoral fractures is to allow full weight bearing as soon as possible, restore patient mobility and function, and reduce hospital stays and the rate of death and medical complications. Some studies indicate that the difference between the costs of the different types of treatment is negligible if the total cost of care is considered; days of hospitalization, rehabilitation, and indirect costs [26–29]. We must consider distal femoral replacement in non-reconstructible cases

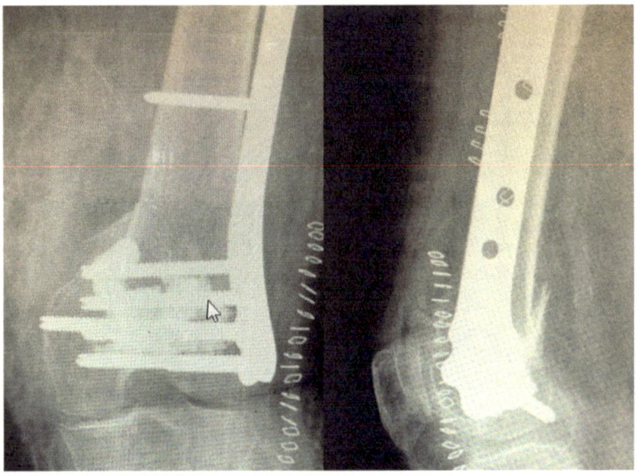

Figure 11.
PMMA augmentation in a distal complex femoral fracture.

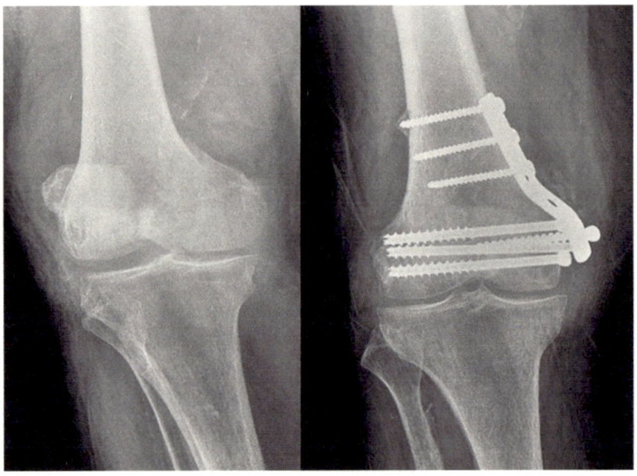

Figure 12.
Hoffa fracture fixed with interfragmentary compression and neutralization plate.

(**Figure 13**) to prevent hardware failure and in periprosthetic fractures without a bone stock for fixation. The two major problems with distal femoral replacement are infection and surgical stress on the patient. We should select our patients properly because the rescue of a distal femoral replacement in an old patient would be catastrophic, and the optimization of the physiological status is mandatory to prevent complications.

Periprosthetic fractures constitute a greater challenge, since the presence of the implant limits bone metabolism and its consolidation capacity, increases the infection rate, we generally work on stiffer knees and, furthermore, the use of retrograde nails is not always possible. In the case we select a locking nails as the method of tratment, it is essential to use as many locking screws in the distal fragment as possible to improve purchase and prevent complications [30].

In these cases, we must be meticulous, study the loads to which the fracture will be subjected, assume long consolidation times, and achieve fixations that are sufficiently rigid to allow early loading (**Figure 14**), while being careful with soft tissue dissection to prevent postoperative complications.

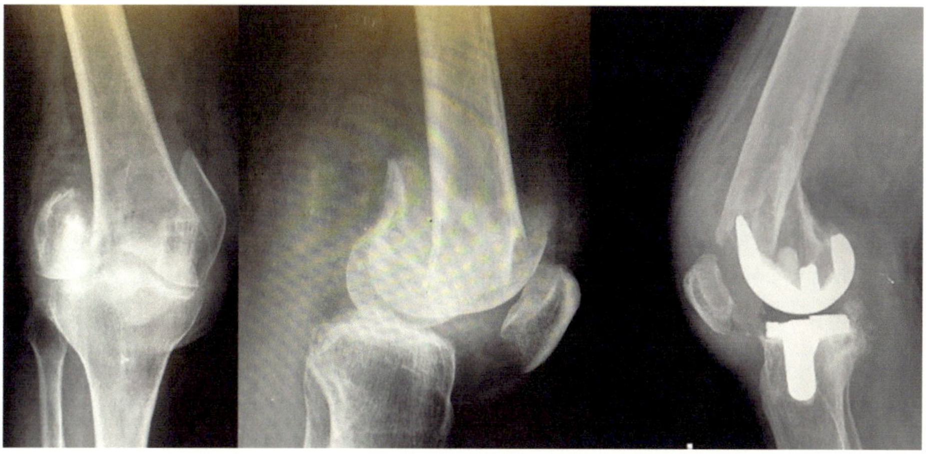

Figure 13.
Situations where a DFR could be an option.

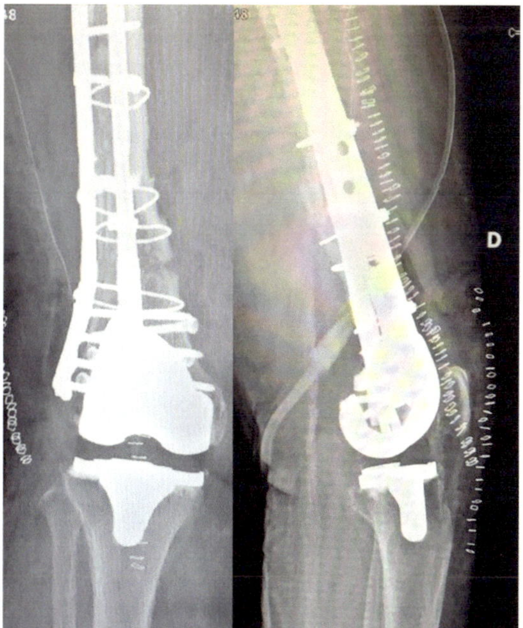

Figure 14.
Rigid bone-plate construct to fix a distal femoral periprosthetic fracture.

7. Complications

Nonunion is the most frequent cause of reoperation in distal femur fractures [31]. Improvements in outcomes have been reported, probably due to "biologic approaches" and implant developments with nonunion rates of 6% [32]. Among the factors that lead to nonunion are metaphyseal comminution, especially medially, malalignment, poor bone quality, and comorbidities that reduce the adequate vascular supply of the bone, such as smoking, diabetes or vascular disease, and inadequate fixation with devices that are too rigid or plates that are too short [31, 33, 34]. Cases of non-septic nonunions in patients with good bone stock should be treated by revision of the implant and bone grafting. In special cases, resorbable methyl methacrylate or tricalcium phosphate cements can be added to "augment" fixation screws in the condylar fragment. Currently, the rate of cure, nonunion, and reoperation is similar between the different fixation methods [18].

Malalignment together with medial comminution are the main factors that predict nonunion [35]. The metaphyseal location with a predominance of cancellous bone predisposes to comminution of the fracture site, even with low-energy trauma. This leads to failure of the constructs with a varus collapse, especially if a lateral fixed angle plate is used [14]. In case of medial comminution greater than 2 cm, it is recommended to add a medial support by means of a "strut allograft," a support plate medial or intramedullary nailing [31, 36]. It should be added that misalignment greater than 5–10 degrees can affect the biomechanics of the knee, conditioning the compartmental overload of the knee [37].

Deep infection rates of around 2.7% have been reported, considerably low when compared to those reported in the 1960 literature [14, 34, 38]. This complication requires meticulous debridement, culture, and appropriate antibiotic therapy. If the fracture allows, it may be appropriate to remove the fixation material. An infection with abscess formation should be "packed open" and some authors recommend the use of vacuum-assisted close therapy, but this point is controversial in the set of an infection [14, 37]. They are generally treated for 3–12 weeks with specific antibiotic therapy [27]. Given implant loosening and recalcitrant infection, removal of the implant and external fixation should be considered. Lower rates of infection have been shown with minimally invasive approaches than with open approaches [39].

Knee stiffness is the most common complication resulting from the initial trauma and surgical exposure. The effect of both is multiplied by prolonged immobilization depending on the surgical technique, which is why early mobilization is necessary, mainly in the case of intra-articular fractures.

8. Conclusions

Distal femoral fractures are challenging, and we should differentiate the two most common types of injuries: younger patients with high-energy fractures with comminution, which should be addressed with dual fixation to prevent varus stress and nonunion, and femoral fractures in the elderly, where the use of augmentation may solve purchase fixation and prevent failure while favoring early weight bearing.

Conflict of interest

The authors declare no conflict of interest.

Author details

Renzo Reyes[1], María González-Alonso[1], Samer Amhaz-Escanlar[1], Alberto De Castro[1], Jesús Pino-Mínguez[1,2] and Alberto Jorge-Mora[1,2]*

1 University Hospital of Santiago de Compostela, Santiago de Compostela, Spain

2 University of Santiago de Compostela, Santiago de Compostela, Spain

*Address all correspondence to: alberto.agustin.jorge.mora@sergas.es

References

[1] Court-Brown CM, Caesar B. Epidemiology of adult fractures: A review. Injury. 2006;**37**(8):691-697

[2] Elsoe R, Ceccotti AA, Larsen P. Population-based epidemiology and incidence of distal femur fractures. International Orthopaedics. 2018;**42**(1):191-196

[3] Martinet O, Cordey J, Harder Y, Maier A, Buhler M, Barraud GE. The epidemiology of fractures of the distal femur. Injury. 2000;**31**(Suppl. 3):C62-C63

[4] Roy D, Ramski D, Malige A, Beck M, Jeffers K, Brogle P. Injury patterns and outcomes associated with fractures of the native distal femur in adults. European Journal of Trauma and Emergency Surgery. 2021;**47**(4):1123-1128

[5] Larsen P, Ceccotti AA, Elsoe R. High mortality following distal femur fractures: A cohort study including three hundred and two distal femur fractures. International Orthopaedics. 2020;**44**(1):173-177

[6] Ebraheim NA, Kelley LH, Liu X, Thomas IS, Steiner RB, Liu J. Periprosthetic distal femur fracture after Total knee arthroplasty: A systematic review. Orthopaedic Surgery. 2015;**7**(4):297-305

[7] Della Rocca GJ, Leung KS, Pape HC. Periprosthetic fractures: Epidemiology and future projections. Journal of Orthopaedic Trauma. 2011;**25**(Suppl. 2): S66-S70

[8] Buckley R, Mohanty K, Malish D. Lower limb malrotation following MIPO technique of distal femoral and proximal tibial fractures. Injury. 2011;**42**(2):194-199

[9] Rüedi TP, Murphy WM, Colton CL, Fackelman GE, Harder Y. AO principles of fracture management. Thieme Stuttgart. 2000;**2**:473-485

[10] Gangavalli AK, Nwachuku CO. Management of Distal Femur Fractures in adults: An overview of options. The Orthopedic Clinics of North America. 2016;**47**(1):85-96

[11] Paley D. Principles of deformity correction. Springer Science & Business Media. Berlin, Heidelberg: Springer; 2002

[12] Rouviere H, Delmas A. Human anatomy. Vol. 412. España: Elsevier; 2000. p. 413

[13] Maslow JI, Collinge CA. Course of the femoral artery in the mid- and distal thigh and implications for medial approaches to the distal femur: A CT angiography study. The Journal of the American Academy of Orthopaedic Surgeons. 2019;**27**(14):e659-ee63

[14] Ricci WM, Mehta S. Orthopaedic Knowledge Update®: Trauma. AAOS EEUU: Lippincott Williams & Wilkins; 2021

[15] Levy BA, Zlowodzki MP, Graves M, Cole PA. Screening for extermity arterial injury with the arterial pressure index. The American Journal of Emergency Medicine. 2005;**23**(5):689-695

[16] Meinberg EG, Agel J, Roberts CS, Karam MD, Kellam JF. Fracture and dislocation classification compendium—2018. Journal of orthopaedic trauma. 2018;**32**:S1-S10

[17] Onay T, Gulabi D, Colak I, Bulut G, Gumustas SA, Cecen GS. Surgically treated Hoffa fractures with poor long-term functional results. Injury. 2018;**49**(2):398-403

[18] Merino-Rueda LR, Rubio-Saez I, Mills S, Rubio-Suarez JC. Mortality after distal femur fractures in the elderly. Injury. 2021;**52**(Suppl. 4):S71-SS5

[19] Zhang Y, Xing B, Hou X, Li Y, Li G, Han G, et al. Comparison of three methods of Muller type C2 and C3 distal femoral fracture repair. The Journal of International Medical Research. 2021;**49**(5):3000605211015031

[20] Meccariello L, Bisaccia M, Ronga M, Falzarano G, Caraffa A, Rinonapoli G, et al. Locking retrograde nail, non-locking retrograde nail and plate fixation in the treatment of distal third femoral shaft fractures: Radiographic, bone densitometry and clinical outcomes. Journal of Orthopaedics and Traumatology. 2021;**22**(1):33

[21] Reeb AF, Collinge CA, Rodriguez-Buitrago AF, Archdeacon MT, Beltran MJ, Gardner MJ, et al. Analysis of 101 mechanical failures in distal femur fractures treated with 3 generations of Precontoured locking plates. Journal of Orthopaedic Trauma. 2022. [Online ahead of print]

[22] Marchand LS, Todd DC, Kellam P, Adeyemi TF, Rothberg DL, Maak TG. Is the lesser trochanter profile a reliable means of restoring anatomic rotation after femur fracture fixation? Clinical Orthopaedics and Related Research. 2018;**476**(6):1253-1261

[23] Liu JF, Zhou ZF, Hou XD, Chen YX, Zheng LP. Hybrid locked medial plating in dual plate fixation optimizes the healing of comminuted distal femur fractures: A retrospective cohort study. Injury. 2021;**52**(6):1614-1620

[24] Wahnert D, Lange JH, Schulze M, Gehweiler D, Kosters C, Raschke MJ. A laboratory investigation to assess the influence of cement augmentation of screw and plate fixation in a simulation of distal femoral fracture of osteoporotic and non-osteoporotic bone. Bone Joint Journal. 2013;**95-B**(10):1406-1409

[25] Beltran MJ, Gary JL, Collinge CA. Management of distal femur fractures with modern plates and nails: State of the art. Journal of Orthopaedic Trauma. 2015;**29**(4):165-172

[26] Hake ME, Davis ME, Perdue AM, Goulet JA. Modern implant options for the treatment of distal femur fractures. The Journal of the American Academy of Orthopaedic Surgeons. 2019;**27**(19):e867-ee75

[27] Pasurka M, Krinner S, Gelse K. Osteosynthesis or arthroplasty of fractures near the knee joint in geriatric patients - a clinical-economical comparison. Zeitschrift für Orthopädie und Unfallchirurgie. 2020;**158**(3):283-290

[28] Rice OM, Springer BD, Karunakar MA. Acute distal femoral replacement for fractures about the knee in the elderly. The Orthopedic Clinics of North America. 2020;**51**(1):27-36

[29] Tandon T, Tadros BJ, Avasthi A, Hill R, Rao M. Management of periprosthetic distal femur fractures using distal femoral arthroplasty and fixation - comparative study of outcomes and costs. Journal of Clinical Orthopaedic Trauma. 2020;**11**(1):160-164

[30] Toro-Ibarguen A, Moreno-Beamud JA, Porras-Moreno MA, Aroca-Peinado M, Leon-Baltasar JL, Jorge-Mora AA. The number of locking screws predicts the risk of nonunion and reintervention in periprosthetic total knee arthroplasty fractures treated with a nail. European Journal of Orthopaedic Surgery and Traumatology. 2015;**25**(4):661-664

[31] Koso RE, Terhoeve C, Steen RG, Zura R. Healing, nonunion, and re-operation after internal fixation of diaphyseal and distal femoral fractures: A systematic review and meta-analysis. International Orthopaedics. 2018;**42**(11):2675-2683

[32] Ocalan E, Ustun CC, Aktuglu K. Locking plate fixation versus antegrade intramedullary nailing for the treatment of extra-articular distal femoral fractures. Injury. 2019;**50**(Suppl. 3):55-62

[33] Parks C, McAndrew CM, Spraggs-Hughes A, Ricci WM, Silva MJ, Gardner MJ. In-vivo stiffness assessment of distal femur fracture locked plating constructs. Clinical Biomechanics (Bristol, Avon). 2018;**56**:46-51

[34] Rajasekaran RB, Jayaramaraju D, Palanisami DR, Agraharam D, Perumal R, Kamal A, et al. A surgical algorithm for the management of recalcitrant distal femur nonunions based on distal femoral bone stock, fracture alignment, medial void, and stability of fixation. Archives of Orthopaedic and Trauma Surgery. 2019;**139**(8):1057-1068

[35] Peschiera V, Staletti L, Cavanna M, Saporito M, Berlusconi M. Predicting the failure in distal femur fractures. Injury. 2018;**49**(Suppl. 3):S2-S7

[36] Spitler CA, Bergin PF, Russell GV, Graves ML. Endosteal substitution with an intramedullary rod in fractures of the femur. Journal of Orthopaedic Trauma. 2018;**32**(Suppl. 1):S25-SS9

[37] Green DP. Rockwood and Green's Fractures in Adults. EEUU: Lippincott Williams & Wilkins; 2010

[38] Gwathmey FW Jr, Jones-Quaidoo SM, Kahler D, Hurwitz S, Cui Q. Distal femoral fractures: Current concepts. The Journal of the American Academy of Orthopaedic Surgeons. 2010;**18**(10):597-607

[39] von Keudell A, Shoji K, Nasr M, Lucas R, Dolan R, Weaver MJ. Treatment options for distal femur fractures. Journal of Orthopaedic Trauma. 2016;**30**(Suppl. 2): S25-S27

Section 2

New Perspectives

Chapter 7

Perspective Chapter: The Complex Architecture of a Traumatic Brain Injury

Leighton J. Reynolds

Abstract

This is a perspective chapter that explores the crucial importance of understanding the full impact and architecture of a traumatic brain injury, beginning with the conception of a "Shock Trauma." This architecture is followed by the brain/mind architecture of "electrical and chemical disruptions in the brain," the brain/mind architecture of "homeostasis, allostasis, and allostatic load causing further disruptions in brain and mind functioning," and the brain/mind architecture of the "perfect storm" in the brain. Each architecture represents a stage in the toxic, cascading progression of a traumatic brain injury. It is generally not understood that traumatic brain injuries are not static events and that they can quickly become neurodegenerative disease processes, especially if they are not treated. Over time, these Four Architectures fold into one another creating huge challenges for the healing process. The conception of the Four Architectures is well illustrated through the case of a 20 year-old female who suffered a brain hemorrhage at age 7. Unfortunately, no follow-up was considered after a year of treatment. Her case identifies the importance of understanding the toxic, cascading progression of a traumatic brain injury through the Four Architectures, and how serious a condition this can become. Finally, the author discusses how brain injuries are different from all other types of injuries to a person, because of their neurodegenerative nature. And that these injuries need to be understood in a very different light, with a great deal more follow-up.

Keywords: TBI, PTSD, shock trauma, neurovascular coupling, homeostasis, allostasis, allostatic load, CTE, AD, PD, dementia

1. Introduction

A number of authors and articles [1–5] have addressed the conception that "head trauma is the beginning of an ongoing, perhaps lifelong, process that impacts multiple organ systems and may be both disease causative and accelerative (1)." This post-traumatic mortality can include neurological disorders (epilepsy and sleep disorders), neurological diseases (AD, CTE, ALS, PD, and dementia), neuroendocrine disorders (post-traumatic hypopituitarism), psychiatric disorders (schizophrenia and manic/

depression), and non-neurological disorders (sexual dysfunction, incontinence, musculoskeletal dysfunction, and metabolic dysfunction) [1]. This chapter agrees with this conception of the major consequences of a TBI and explains why and how this occurs through an understanding of the Four Architectures of a TBI. I introduce the case of S. as a demonstration of how devastating the consequences of a TBI can be for an individual's life without this understanding.

2. The case of MS. S

S. began working with me when she was 20 years old. At that time, her mother was desperate to find some answers that would explain her daughter's deteriorating condition and her defiant behavior. S. could not sleep at night. And she could not wake up in the morning with any energy or motivation. She was chronically fatigued and would frequently lash out at her mother over "small stuff." She had difficulties with concentration, focus, and attention. Reading and writing for any length of time were out of the question because she became exhausted when attempting either reading or writing for very long. She could barely remain on a computer for 15 minutes. Regarding work and school, S. could not hold down a job, because of the above and she was failing out of school. And probably the worst for her: she was in constant physical pain day in and day out. Later we discovered through a 72-hour EEG, that she was having multiple absence seizures throughout the day. This was not good news! In the meantime, her mother had struggled for years to find answers to what was wrong with her daughter. And no answers were available.

Finally, one June afternoon her mother brought S. in to see me. After sharing her daughter's long list of symptoms, she asked:

"Could her symptoms have anything to do with the accident that happened to her when she was 7-years-old?"

When S. was 7 years old she was thrown off the back of a horse when the horse bolted, and she hit the back of her head on a rock. Her mother explained that she heard screaming and ran back out of the ranch house where she had gone to pick up an item. By the time she reached S. she was lying motionless on the ground, and her eyes had rolled back into her head.

As her mother explained it: "No one wants to see their child like this!"

With the help of their neighbors, S. was airlifted to a nearby trauma center where she underwent emergency surgery for a brain hematoma and a depressed skull fracture. The neurosurgery included the placement of two mental plates. One year later, S. had a second surgery to remove the screws holding the metal plates. During this period, she appeared to have recovered quite nicely.

"Was there any follow-up from there," I asked?

Her Mother replied: "No, not really. No one was paying much attention after that. And our lives moved on."

S.'s mother related she was told that they were lucky the injury was on the occipital lobe and that part of the brain managed mostly vision. She was told that her daughter would be able to have a normal life, but to keep an eye on her vision. Nothing was ever mentioned about looking out for problems with CPS (post-concussion syndrome).

Everything appeared to be normal for S. except for issues around concentrating and organization in school. However, early on S. did express having intense, overwhelming

DOI: http://dx.doi.org/10.5772/intechopen.108554

feelings with her friends during grade school, and often experienced stomach upsets. Unfortunately, her mother did not associate these difficulties with her head injury because of the "good news" prognosis given by S.'s neurologist and the.

supporting medical staff treating her case. But when S. entered her teenage years, she began to display further obvious and more intense behaviors: acting out, impulsive and dangerous behaviors, cutting, threatening suicide, defiance, severe difficulties in school (socially), could not follow a normal sleep pattern, had difficulties with math, reading, and writing, and could not focus for very long on anything. Her mother brought her into treatment where she was labeled severely depressed and ADHD and medicated. But nothing changed. And S. continued to be seen as a "problem child."

S.'s psychological evaluation, done when she was age 15, addressed the fact that S. was performing poorly in school, had difficulty paying attention in school, reported feeling highly anxious and was hearing voices, and had difficulties keeping up with her classmates. She was diagnosed then with: persistent depressive disorder, generalized anxiety disorder, and attention deficit hyperactivity disorder, combined type. Again, there was no mention of any possible connection to her TBI at age 7.

Sadly, this pattern continued into high school and S. ended up not graduating from high school. As her mother looked back on those years, she explained to me that: "This wasn't my child anymore. Where did she go? I didn't know who she was anymore."

What lies ahead in this chapter is the story of S. in the context of the Four Architectures I understand that occur with all traumatic brain injuries. My goal is to "paint the picture" of these Four Architectures as they played out in S.'s case and present the perspective that after a TBI, there is much more that needs to be done. Much more, because a traumatic brain injury is really the beginning of a neurodegenerative disease process in the brain/mind [1–5]. In not following through the progression of a TBI, persons end up in the same situation R. did when she first came to see me. And this is a very difficult place to be as you can see from the above symptomatology R. presented with.

Against this background, S.'s original injury was the following: depressed right parietal skull fracture with underlying parenchymal contusion, subarachnoid hemorrhage, pneumocephalus, and overlying scalp laceration. She received excellent medical care for her injury. However, again, there was no follow-up. The concept of the Four Architectures argues that there is much more to an original traumatic brain injury and that not following through with continued treatment leads to serious consequences. Exactly as S. has been experiencing since elementary school.

3. The Four Architectures

In my experience, all blows to the head follow a similar architecture that, again, does not lead to a good place. Especially, if not recognized, addressed, and treated. Too often, trauma to the brain/mind ends up as Alzheimer's Disease, Parkinson's Disease, MS, ALS, CTE, or dementia in general following the path of the Four Architectures I describe here. And as research is now informing us, trauma to the brain/mind can also lead to serious mental disorders, most notably schizophrenia and manic/depression (bipolar I & II) [4, 5].

S.'s symptomatology unfortunately fits an injury pattern I am seeing too often because of misunderstandings and misconceptions of the cascading course of a traumatic brain injury. Her Spect Scan, done when she was age 20, demonstrated small scattered focal areas of predominately mild hypoperfusion in five different areas of her brain (September 18, 2020). Again, her case illustrates so well the consequences of not treating this cascading progression of a TBI. Her Spect Scan is proof that her original injury at age 7 was not a static event. Rather, it was the beginning of a serious neurodegenerative disease process.

Why am I using the word "architecture" to describe this cascading, neurodegenerative process in the brain/mind/body? One of the definitions of the word architecture (in addition to the standard definition of the word as the art and practice of designing and constructing building) is "the complex or carefully designed structure of something." An example would be: "The chemical or electrical structure of the brain." I will be exploring this conceptualization with the outline of Architecture Two. For now, I am referring to the complex architecture (structure and design) that follows trauma to the entire brain/mind/body.

Architecture One following a TBI can best be described and understood as a "Shock Trauma." A Shock Trauma is an automatic defense mechanism that helps protect the brain and the body from further damage. This protection process is accompanied by a range of physical and psychological symptoms that include [6]:

- Numbness
- Confusion
- Dissociation
- Dizziness
- Rapid Heart Rate

In the literature I explored, this "alarm response" (see the work of Hans Seyle dating back to the 1930s) usually lasts for seconds to minutes. But in my experience, if this architecture is not adequately addressed, it continues to proceed in the brain/mind/body as the person's homeostatic balance attempts to restore itself, too often unsuccessfully. What I have yet to find in the literature is any widespread recognition that this recovery process in the brain does not in fact come to a quick halt. Instead, there are many factors influencing the individual's recovery from a shock trauma. Not the least of which is the patient's personality, character, developmental history, and prior illnesses and diseases. And over time, this rebalancing attempt, if uncorrected, will result in a further deterioration process in the mind/brain/body [7].

The specifics of the physical process of a Shock Trauma include [6]:

- A sudden decrease in blood flow
- An irregular heart beat
- Lightheadedness
- Nausea

- Muscle tension
- Difficulty moving or functioning at all
- Unconsciousness
- The psychological symptoms include:
- Brain fog
- Numbness
- Disconnection from reality
- Denial about what just happened
- Withdrawal into oneself
- Increased anxiety and depression
- Panic
- Confusion and disorientation
- An inability to concentrate and focus
- Difficulties coping with the immediate emotions and memories

Again, these symptoms are all related to the body's attempts to rebalance itself but are seldom viewed this way. All the patients I have worked with over the past 6 years who have immediately gone to the ER have received an MRI (which did not show any damage to the brain), and they were sent home and told to rest for at least a week before returning to their "regular" lives. The perceptive that something is already going on in their brain/mind, which is potentially very dangerous, is totally missing.

One could logically suspect that this initial shock to the brain/mind/body would be a short-term process. The brain/mind/body restores itself and the person's life appears to have gone back to normal. After all, the person does appear to be normal in every respect. However, this is not what I have witnessed on too many occasions. In S.'s case, she appeared to be developmentally fine moving forward with her life as a normal kid would. But in fact, this was not to be the case for her. As her mother later shared with me looking back, by her teenage years S. was already becoming problematic. But no one really.

understood why. I note that the evaluations done for S. at that time were only psychological. There was no consideration of what might be going on in her brain as a result of the accident that occurred when she was 7 years old.

Note that all brain trauma (including a TBI, a stroke, infections, disease processes, and tumors) is traumatic to an individual. And further, we cannot separate the individual person from their injury. Trauma is always subjective in part and is often less indicative about the actual event and more about the ways a person interprets the experience and makes meaning of their traumatic experience. I note that mental processing will affect the person's physical recovery [8, 9]. And that this fact will influence the course of all Four Architectures. And yes, these psychological factors will show up on evaluations. But they are not the entire story of what a patient (like S.) is dealing with.

Looking further into Architecture One, there are basically two overarching kinds of shock traumas. Dissociative shock traumas occur when a person disconnects from themselves and others around them to reduce the amount of stimulation they must deal with daily [6]. This is an automatic, unconscious process, during which the person often feels disconnected from reality, often develops memory loss for the event (or events over time), and can manifest as a long-term dissociative disorder.

The other variation of a shock trauma is medical (although I believe that the physical and the mental interact as one). With hypovolemic shock traumas, there can be severe blood and fluid loss making it difficult for the heart to pump blood causing vital organs in the body to lose functionality. With distributive shock traumas, the.

result is abnormalities with the blood vessels that interfere with the distribution of blood in the body, possibly leading to low blood pressure and collapse. With cardiac shock traumas, there is a heart attack, and the heart is unable to pump blood to the body. And finally, there are neurogenic shock traumas when the brain and spinal cord are injured. Damage to the nervous system will also interfere with and block normal blood flow [6]. None of this is good and puts the person's life at risk for brain/mind problems in the future. And again, especially if not addressed.

In my experience, all of this occurs as the mind/body attempts to, again, rebalance itself in the face of huge disruptions to its homeostatic balance. I note that the most important function of our brains is not thinking, but rather survival [10]. Hence any trauma to the brain threatens our very survival. Nor, in my experience, does this rebalancing process necessarily subside in a short period of time. It can literally go on for years, especially if not addressed.

Finally, note that work is being done to better understand the immediate effects of a "shock trauma," through an understanding of the concept of Neurovascular Coupling [11–14]. I will be exploring neurovascular coupling further in Architecture Two as a major cause of disruptions to brain/mind functioning following a TBI. And I note the authors' statement that: "Given the difficulty of rapid detection, mTBI poses a particular challenge to public health because repeated injuries such as concussions have a cumulative effect on brain health" [11] (045007–1). The use of the phrase "cumulative effect on brain health" is why I believe understanding and treating the Four Architectures is so important, illustrated so well through S.'s case.

Architecture Two addresses disruptions to the electrical and chemical signals in the brain/mind. Literally, that makes us human! As TBI research is demonstrating, "There is increasing evidence that TBIs promotes the accumulation, misfolding, and aggregation of multiple abnormal proteins associated with neurodegeneration including tau, B-amyloid, a-synuclein, and tar DNA binding 43 proteins" [2] (p.9). And "A single moderate to severe TBI with LOC is associated with a two-to-fourfold increased risk of dementia in later life" [2, 15]. Note here that: "It is increasingly clear that TBI is a process and not a static injury, and that prolonged symptoms in TBI survivors represent functional and structural damage in the brain" ([2], p. 21). One of the brain systems most affected by this architecture is the neurovascular coupling system in the brain. NVC refers to the important connection between the nerve cells in the brain (the neurons) and their vascular (blood) supply. This is the source of energy that allows the brain/mind to both work and function properly. This coupling between the neurons and their vascular supply controls blood flow in the brain giving the neurons their energy to send and receive messages. Without the nutrients and oxygen regulated by NVC, the brain/mind cannot function adequately. And once the brain/mind has been damaged through a TBI (or other insults), it is very difficult to re-establish this important coupling. This results in the wide variety of symptoms we see with a TBI.

I have no information that would indicate S. was treated for a "shock trauma" following her accident. Although she did recover reasonably quickly following her neurosurgery. My concern is that by not fully addressing the effects of a "shock trauma" and doing long-term follow-up appointments, something very important is being missed.

"And what kinds of symptoms are you experiencing now, S.?"

"I don't function at all anymore. I mostly stay in my room all day, because I just don't have any energy anymore."

"And you're in constant pain?"

"Yes, I don't even want to get out of bed in the morning."

"Because of the pain?"

"What's the point if you're in constant pain!"

In S.'s case, this is all a result of long-term PCS (post-concussion syndrome) that had gone unrecognized and untreated. When the brain/mind is injured and unable to regulate blood flow to the neurons through NVC, the result is chronic fatigue and exhaustion, daily headaches, slow thinking, heavy brain fog, confusion, disorientation, memory loss, chronic sleep deprivation, and an inability to concentrate or focus on much of anything. This was unfortunately S. to a "T."

Too often this entire process goes unrecognized (and hence untreated) because vascular damage to the brain does not show up on an MRI (which is looking at structural issues in the brain). Standard structural clinical neuroimaging studies show no abnormal findings for the majority of PCS patients. For these patients, the damage is caused by cerebrovascular dysregulation and neuronal dysfunction [12]. Brain imaging studies using fMRI or Spect Scan technology are far more useful in demonstrating this kind of damage in the brain. "In short, it is becoming increasingly clear that NVC alterations, along with cerebrovascular reactivity (CVR) disruptions and autonomic nervous system (ANS) dysregulation play a significant role in PCS sequelae" ([10], p.1).

Sadly, there is more damage done to the brain beyond disruptions with neurovascular coupling (as damaging as this is). The mechanical forces involved in brain trauma (acceleration and deceleration linear, rotational, forces associated with blast injuries, blunt impact, and penetration by a projectile) cause direct damage to the neurons, dendrites, glia, and blood vessels in focal, multifocal, and/or diffuse patterns in the brain, and initiate a dynamic series of complex cellular, inflammatory, mitochondrial, neurochemical, and metabolic alterations ([2], pp. 2–3). While the immediate neurologic damage from primary traumatic forces is usually not alterable, the secondary damage produced by a cascading series of events does have the potential to be reversed. It is this cascading series of events that result in Architecture Two. For more information about reversing the secondary damage from a TBI see my forthcoming "Listening To The Brain" with Cambridge Scholars Publishing (2023).

Within Architecture Two of a TBI, I reiterate what I have stated above, because I believe this is so important to recognize that a TBI is not a static neurological insult to the brain/mind. It is now clear that a TBI can trigger progressive neurodegenerative damage leading to various forms of dementia (Alzheimer's Disease, Parkinson's Disease, ALS, Lewy body disease, CTE, and MS). Cognitive impairments with these diseases include memory loss, speed processing problems (which I find with all my

TBI patients), and executive functioning decline proceed long after the initial injury. Increasing epidemiological evidence demonstrates the links between head injury and an increased risk of dementia [16]. And exactly what is the link involved here between a TBI and an increasing path toward dementia of some type?

In a rather unusual manner (the brain is a different animal), the flow of the brain (the interactions between the various networks in the brain) begins to break down as literally broken pieces of the nerve cells (the neurons) and the supporting glia cells begin to clump together in a toxic process that cascades through the brain/mind. This leads to a host of symptoms that are at once invisible and very damaging. I believe this process is what is currently considered to be PCS. The culprits most identified in this cascading, degenerative processes are abnormal tau amyloid beta, and TDP-43. "The neurotoxicity of these pathogenic proteins (e.g., cis-P-tau) contributing directly to neuronal loss seen after injury is a potential link between acute and chronic of post-TBI changes" ([4], p. 1221). In my experience, there is a direct link here demonstrated so clearly in [4] (see Open Access: Understanding Neurodegeneration, p. 1225).

Architecture Two, then, addresses many factors all leading in the direction that the normal functioning of the brain/mind has now become toxic. And if not recognized and treated, will continue toward some form of dementia. I note that a person's entire existence is at risk when there are severe disruptions to the brain's electrical and chemical systems. This is how neurons talk to one another and give us our life force! But now, due to unrecognized and untreated "shock trauma" that the body/mind experienced, there is a cascading process of toxic build-up in the brain/mind. This is the concern of Architecture Two, which was initiated through a "shock trauma" that has gone unrecognized and hence untreated.

Architecture Three involves the following:

In my experience, medicine, psychology, and the legal system do not pay enough attention to the very important concept of Homeostasis. Homeostasis references the constant need our bodies, and our minds have, to maintain the balance of our physiology, our biochemistry, our neurology, and our psychology. Homeostasis is how we sustain our lives! The related concept of Allostasis addresses the moment-by-moment changes our bodies and our minds are constantly creating to keep us in the range of homeostatic balance. And where is the master switch for this crucial process to every individual on the planet? Yes, our brains accomplish this feat every moment of our existence. But again, our question is what happens when the brain is injured? When there are huge disruptions in a person's ability to function effectively in their everyday lives because their homeostatic balance is in question. Then, these individuals cannot function normally!

As noted in Architecture Two, the toxic processes cascading through the brain/mind following the disruptions in brain functions from a TBI are not just isolated aspects of the brain. The person's entire being is affected. Why? Because when the Master Switch (the brain) of everyone's existence is damaged, the processes of Homeostasis and Allostasis are affected on a very large scale. And this is what accounts for the wide range of symptoms that brain-injured persons experience. We are now in the midst of Architecture Three, when the brain/mind/body is working overtime to maintain homeostatic balance, and the allostatic resources to do so are simply not there. The energy necessary (driven by processes in the brain) to restore homeostatic balance and maintain body budgeting is not available because the master switch in the brain has been damaged [17]. This is what causes the pervasive symptomatology we encounter with all brain injuries (especially when not treated). Consider that there are no other medical problems that are so pervasive in an individual's life. Broken arms, broken legs, kidney infections, IBS problems, and skin disorders for example do not affect the entire body in the manner that an injury to the brain will do. Yet we recognize so little about this!

The third consideration we need to pay attention to here as part of Architecture Three is allostatic load [17]. The primary hormonal mediators of the stress response in the body are glucocorticoids and catecholamines. They have both protective and damaging effects on the body. In the short run sphere, they are essential for adaptation, the maintenance of Homeostasis, and the survival of the mind/body/brain through Allostasis. But over time, these managing processes exact a cost (Allostatic Load) that can begin and accelerate disease processes. The paradox here is the systems that automatically respond to stressful episodes in all of us, the autonomic nervous system and adrenocortical system in the body, are indeed protectors of the body in the short run. But over time, they cause damage and accelerate diseases in the mind/brain/body. Specifically, allostatic load refers to the price the mind/body/brain pays for being forced to adapt to adverse physical, psychological, and/or environmental situations. Allostatic load represents both the presence of too much stress and/or the inefficient operation of the stress hormonal response system ([17], p. 114).

An additional (and major) concern of Architecture Three is the role of increasing demands on the brain/mind/body following a TBI.

Demands on the brain, for any reason (no matter how small), demand energy, and as a consequence take energy away from the healing process and increase allostatic load [17]. And as noted above, increases in allostatic load led to further damage and injury to the person struggling with a TBI. I note that for all my patients, as they begin to resume their normal activities, they begin to experience continuing episodes of chronic fatigue. Thus, it is very difficult to "get ahead" with an injury to the brain unless there are major opportunities for rest and healing.

And finally, not to further complicate the cascading, progression of a TBI, there is Architecture Four, the "perfect storm" in the brain [18, 19]. We know that brain injuries slow down the processing of this person's world, internal and external. I have had to learn in working with TBI patients, to give them plenty of "room" and time to process their thoughts and feelings and respond during sessions. I likened this experience for the patient to the running of a slow computer. Because either something is wrong with the computer or it is out of date with its processing speed and power. Does this cause problems for persons experiencing a TBI, in a modern culture that is now always moving exponentially? Yes! At the same time, all brain injuries are traumatizing experiences for that individual and therefore cases of PTSD. What does PTSD do in the brain? It speeds things up as the HPA axis works to cope with a mind/body/brain that is under seize (Howard Weiner). In my experience, trauma is at the root of all PTSD issues. And what could be more traumatizing than "losing your brain/mind," because it will affect every aspect of your life.

PTSD is the brain/mind/body's response to being traumatized (when the event overwhelms the person's ability to cope). The symptomatology of PTSD includes [19]:

- Reliving the trauma through flashbacks, hallucinations, nightmares, and memories about the incident.

- Avoiding persons, places, or things that remind the person of the incident, incidents.

- Excessive arousal including being easily startled and frightened, increasing on the alert and on guard for danger, random fits of rage, easily irritated, visible hatred, self-destructive behavior with drugs and ETOH, difficulties with sleep, and an inability to concentrate and focus in all aspects of daily life.

- Intrusive thoughts from distressing and guilty feelings.

- Further symptoms include flat affect, feeling detached from life, a lack of interest in daily life, difficulties experiencing positive emotions, emotional numbness, suicidal ideation, and feeling hopeless about returning to a normal life.

"What's your day-to-day life like S.?"

"I don't really do much. I'm always tired and in pain, which is really no fun!"

"Are you able to read, write, watch TV, see a movie?"

"Not really, I mostly veg every day. I don't have any energy, and if I do something, I always pay for it and end up sleeping a lot."

"Do you feel hopeless about all of this?"

"I don't see anything getting any better. What do you expect. And yes, I do feel suicidal from time to time, because nothing ever seems to get better!"

Architecture Four addresses the fact that there are now clashing forces operating in the brain/mind/body. A TBI slows things down while PTSD speeds things up. Where is the good news here? No wonder so many TBI patients feel like they are going crazy. Then how does anyone cope with a brain/mind/body that is experiencing these clashing events?

See the following references for further details describing the neurodegenerative disease processes that catalyze the development of the Four Architectures. And note that the Four Architectures are the brain/mind's complex response to a traumatic injury [20–26].

4. Discussion

Why am I using the concept of "Architectures" to explain the cascading progression of a TBI? Because these "Architectures" represent the brain's responses to damage, and over time they fold into one another. Further, this damage, over time, will cause huge disruptions in the active flow of the brain/mind/body. It is a neurodegenerative disease process that is causing a cascading, toxic effect in the brain, and by connecting the mind and the body. Since our brains are built to control and ensure our survival (not just thinking which is of course a major part of our survival), damage to the brain is a threat to the person's very day-to-day survival [10]. In my private practice over the past 6 years, I have seen the clear results of how damaging this cascading, neurodegenerative process can be.

Here is a summary of the information supporting the conception of a neurodegenerative disease process in S.'s brain. Her original accident occurred in October of 2007 when she was 7 years old.

S.'s psychological evaluation was done in 2015 (noted above) to address her ongoing behavioral problems. Sadly, nothing about the brain was included, and despite efforts to help S. nothing changed.

Her MRI brain without contrast (July 13, 2020) concluded that there was a focus of cortical and adjacent white matter encephalomalacia [27] that involved the parietal occipital lobe. And that this may represent a focus on cortical contusional injury, or previous intraparenchymal hemorrhage in view of the patient's history.

Her EEG report of 7/21/2020 concluded that her EEG was abnormal and that this abnormal activity was suggestive of a generalized seizure disorder.

Her qSPECT (Spect Scan) of 9/18/2020 concluded that this was an abnormal brain SPECT demonstrating scattered, small focal areas of predominately mild hypoperfusion in five different areas of the brain. I believe these five areas of hypoperfusion are what account for the wide range of symptoms S. is experiencing that are so disabling in her life.

The current list of symptoms that S. lists are quite pervasive indicating huge disruptions in her attempts at Homeostatic Balance (see Architecture Three above). These include:

Difficulties with anger management, blurred vision, confusion and disorientation, following instructions, integrating information, learning new things, concentration and focus, short and long-term memory, and decreased judgment.

Balance problems, increased irritability, low frustration tolerance, mood swings, insomnia, nightmares and sleep paralysis, increased depression and anxiety including suicidal ideation, panic attacks, and paranoia.

Chronic fatigue, headaches, pain, racing thoughts, sensitivity to light, sound, and touch, ringing in the ears, and trauma flashbacks.

Among the patients I have worked with over the past 6 years, this huge range of symptoms is the norm. And when you look at the Four Architectures that fold into one another it is easier to understand how this is happening.

My goal in writing this chapter is to open the door to a more complete understanding of this very complex and complicated process that follows from an injury to the brain. My hope is that this chapter will help to initiate further research, understanding, and treatment of traumatic brain injuries.

I close this chapter with two quotes I believe resonate with my conception of the Four Architectures and points us in the direction of the research, understanding, and TBI treatment we need to focus on:

"Previously, TBI has generally been viewed as producing a static neurological insult. However, it is now clear that it can trigger progressive neurodegeneration and dementia. Cognitive impairments such as memory loss, processing speed problems and executive dysfunction are common, and some survivors experience cognitive decline long after injury, in part due to the development of dementia" ([4], p. 1221).

"Advances in the understanding of the neuropathophysiology of TBI suggest that these forces initiate an elaborate and complex array of cellular and subcellular events related to alterations in Ca++ homeostasis and signaling. Furthermore, there is a fairly predictable profile of brain regions that are impacted by neurotrauma and the related events. This profile of brain damage accurately predicts the.

acute and chronic sequelae that TBI survivors suffer from, although there is enough variation to suggest that individual differences such as genetic polymorphisms and factors governing resiliency play a role in modulating outcome" ([28], p. 1).

In my experience, all blows to the head are in some manner insults and disruptions to neurological functioning on some (sometimes many) levels. Accordingly, we need to research this subject in much more depth! (See the research on 12-year-old hockey players in Canada who were asymptomatic following a concussion, but brain damage was clearly visible on follow-up brain imaging.) [29, 30].

Author details

Leighton J. Reynolds
Treatment and Tools for Trauma, Greater Los Angeles, CA, USA

*Address all correspondence to: leightonj@sbcglobal.net

References

[1] Masel BE, DeWitt DS. Traumatic brain Injury: A disease process, not an event. Journal of Neurotrauma. 2010;**27**:1529-1540

[2] McKee AC, Daneshvar DH. The neuropathology of traumatic brain Injury. Handbook of Clinical Neurology. 2015;**127**:45-66

[3] Kemp S, Goulding P, Spencer J, Mitchell AJ. Case study: Unusually rapid and severe cognitive deterioration after mild traumatic brain Injury. Brain Injury. 2005;**19**(14):1269-1276

[4] Graham NSN, Sharp DJ. Understanding neurodegeneration after traumatic brain Injury: From mechanisms to clinical trials in dementia. Neurology, Neurosurgery & Psychiatry. 2019;**90**:1221-1233

[5] Ashman TA, Gordon WA, Cantor JB, Hibbard MR. Neurobehavioral consequences traumatic brain Injury. The Mount Sinai Journal of Medicine. 2006;**73**(7):999-1005

[6] Sanjana Gupta. What is Traumatic Shock. 2022. Available from: https://www.VeryWellMind.com/Traumatic-Shock-Definition-Symptoms-Causes-and-Treatment (5242269)

[7] Williams R. Tau pathology present decades after a single brain Injury. Science Transitional Medicine. 2019;**11**:eaaw1993

[8] Molaie AM, Maguire J. Neuroendocrine abnormalities following traumatic brain Injury: An important contributor to neuropsychiatric sequelae. Frontiers in Endocrinology. 2018;**9**:176

[9] Ashman TA, Gordon WA, Cantor JB, Hibbard MR. Neurobehavioral consequences of traumatic brain Injury. The Mount Sinai Journal of Medicine. 2006;**73**(7):999-1005

[10] Lisa Feldman Barrett. 7 ½ Lessons about the Brain. Boston: Houghton Mifflin Harcourt; 2020

[11] Jang H, Huang S, Hammer DX, Wang L, Rafi H, Ye M, et al. Alterations in neurovascular Coupling following acute traumatic brain Injury. Neurophotonics. 2017;**4**(4): 045007

[12] Allen MD, Epps CT. Neurovascular coupling: A unifying theory for post-concussion syndrome treatment and functional neuroimaging. Journal of Neurology and Neurophysiology. 2017;**8**(6):1000454

[13] Watts ME, Pocock R, Claudianos C. Brain energy and oxygen metabolism: Emerging role in Normal function and disease. Frontiers in Molecular Neuroscience. 2018;**11**:216

[14] Falkowska A, Gutowska I, Goschorska M, Nowacki P, Chlubek D, Baranowska-Bosiacka I. Energy metabolism of the brain, including the cooperation between astrocytes and neurons, especially in the context of glycogen metabolism. International Journal of Molecular Sciences. 2015;**16**:25959-25981

[15] Ryback R. Traumatic Brain Injury: The Invisible Illness (a Single Concussion Can Change your Life). Psychology Today; 2016

[16] Camandola S, Mattson MP. Brain metabolism in health, aging, and neurodegeneration. The EMBO Journal. 2017;**36**:1474-1492

[17] McEwen BS. Allostasis and Allostatic load: Implications for Neuropsychopharmacology. Neuropsychopharmacology. 2000;**22**(2):108-124

[18] Marilyn Lash MSW, TBI and PTSD: Navigating the Perfect Storm, Brain Injury Journey Magazine, Issue #1, 2013

[19] Bryan R. Post-traumatic stress disorder vs traumatic brain Injury. Dialogues in Clinical Neuroscience. 2011;**13**(3):251-262

[20] Mike McRae. Just One Head Injury Could Be Enough to Tangle Proteins in Your Brain. 2019. Available from: https://www.sciencealert.com/one-head-injury-could-be-enough-to-create-the-protein-tangles-in-your-brain

[21] Do Carmo S, Spillantini MG, Cuello AC. Tau pathology in neurological disorders. Frontiers in Neurology. 2021;**12**:754669

[22] Faden AI, Loane DJ, Injury CNATB. Alzheimer disease, chronic traumatic encephalopathy, or persistent Neuroinflammation? Neurotherapeutics. 2015;**12**:143-150

[23] Emily Lunardo. Encephalomalacia: Definition, causes, types, symptoms, and treatment. 2017. Available from: https://belmarrahealth.com/encephalomalacia-causes-types-treatment

[24] Roman Hlatky MD, Alex B, Valadka MD, Claudia S. Intracranial hypertension and cerebral ischemia after severe traumatic brain Injury. Neurosurgical Focus. 2003;**14**(4):2

[25] Pasley BN, Freeman RD, Coupling N. Scholarpedia. 2008;**3**(3):5340

[26] Alina Fong. What You Need to Know About TBI Symptoms and Treatment. 2020. Available from: https://www.cognitivefxusa.com/traumatic-brain-injury-long-term-effect-and-treatment

[27] Encephalomalacia: Definition, Causes, Types, Symptoms, and Treatment. Available from: https://www.belmarrahealth.com/encephalomalacia-causes-types-treatment

[28] Thomas W. McAllister, Neurobiological consequences of traumatic brain Injury, dialogues Clinical Neuroscience. 2011;**13**(3):287-300

[29] Emery C. Concussions Affect 1 in 10 Youth Athletes every Year. Here's What Needs to Change. Calgary, Canada: University of Calgary; 2020

[30] Charles T, Victoria B, Jin Ma. Persisting concussion symptoms from bodychecking: Unrecognized toll in boys ice hockey. Published online. Cambridge University Press; 2022. pp. 1-9